A Christian's Mental Health Guide

For Missionaries, Pastors, & Other Christians Too

By Don Mingo

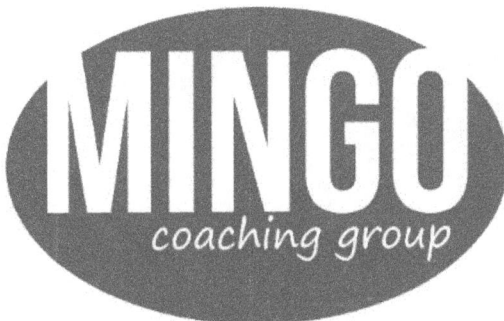

Table of Contents

Acknowledgements

First, gratitude finds limitless boundaries with my Kathy. These past forty-plus years, we've walked this journey together. You've never flinched as we've faced our trials together. Your love is a quality that I've never doubted.

To my family, you make my life complete. Your love, support, and understanding are beyond what few experience.

To my friends in the Mental Health profession, Dr. Mary Cotton, Jane Simmons, Dr. Brian Feldhaus, and Rebeka Whitley, thank you for your input, suggestions, and recommendations.

The many who proofread the manuscript of this book. Thank you for all the suggestions and corrections, bringing this book to a finished work. Thank you, Daniel, my son, for designing another brilliant cover for my book.

Thank you for the much-appreciated editing help from Sarah Odom and Marla Renee Stanley. You were brutally compassionate. Thank you for your corrections, criticisms, and rewrites.

Thank you for the help and encouragement from many of you who make up the Church and for accompanying me on my often perilous journey.

Most of all, I thank God that in the weakest of our weaknesses, there is a purpose to be found. Sometimes, in our feeblest of moments, Christ becomes strongest in our lives. 2 Corinthians 12:9-10

Last, to my brother Bob, who suffered more than anyone I've known. Your body is now free of FSHD Muscular Dystrophy. You'll never hurt again. You were the most positive and thankful person I've ever known. Thanks for encouraging me in my struggles as I learn to deal with this disease.

Preface

The 'A' in *A Christian's Guide to Mental Health* is me. These are some thoughts jotted down over the years while struggling with my own mental health.

What follows is a culmination of dealing with the ravages of PTSD in my life. PTSD affects so much more than just the individual suffering from it. Studying everything out there on how to manage its effects and seeing trauma therapists for protracted sessions, I began learning how to tame this physical injury to the brain.

A new foe joined the battle recently; Facioscapulohumeral Muscular Dystrophy. They refer to this ailment as a 'muscle-wasting disease.' That's an accurate description of what's happening to my body.

Now, we are fighting a war on two fronts. Kathy, my companion, friend, and lover of forty-three years, never flinches. Our sons and their families provide caring support that few experience.

I'm lucky. Blessed.

Gratitude is rooted in optimism.[1]

My thoughts, observations, and personal practices offered in the following pages transpired through attempts at self-preservation. While trying to find answers for the traumatic images buried in my brain from decades of child abuse, missionary service in my adult years, and physical brain injury, this guide developed.

The practices here have helped me. Perhaps they'll also help you in your journey.

Preface

I am not a therapist, professional counselor, or certified mental health professional. What I am is a missionary, pastor, person, and Christ-follower who's battled with my mental health for years, and now a chronic debilitating genetic, physical disease that kept upon me these last ten years. This is just a personal map to navigate my own mental health journey. Glean what you may. Dismiss what you don't like. Take what you can use.

While much of my guide focuses on mental health from a cross-cultural worker's perspective—I was a missionary for over twenty years—you will also find the following pages, which include pastors, those in Christian ministry, and other Christians. My goal is to share with you guideposts developed for my own mental health.

Here's the truth: Pastors, missionaries, and other Christians suffer from the same mental health issues as those outside the church. We've just learned to become proficient at denying it. In trying to save face, we sometimes lose ourselves.

May this guide encourage you to assess and deal with your mental health, seeing Christ in every step you take.

In trying to save face, we sometimes lose ourselves.

It's not so crucial that you agree or disagree with me on a specific point. I'm sharing my thoughts, considerations, and the many possibilities for improving mental health. May this guide encourage you to assess your own mental health and deal with it, seeing Christ in every step you take.

> He *comforts us in all our troubles* so that *we can comfort others.* When they are troubled, we will be able to give them the same comfort God has given us.
>
> 2 Corinthians 1:4 Emphasis Mine

He who is in you is greater than he who is in the world.

1 John 4:4 NKJV

Please make sure you consult your doctor, mental health professional, counselor, or therapist before making any changes in managing your mental health.

Trigger Warning: *In the following pages, topics such as self-harm, abuse, assault, trauma, and suicide will be discussed.*

Reader discretion is advised.

Guideposts

AS A YOUNG TEENAGE BOY, my mom sent us to Youth Retreats every summer way up in Willow River, Minnesota. Now, it wasn't that far from home, mind you, but for two boys traveling three hours in a chartered bus in the early 70s, well now, that was quite an adventure. Paying for that experience was different, as my mother had little income to provide for such luxuries.

Every year while snow was still on the ground, my brother and I entered a competition at Jerry Gamble's Boy's Club to see who could sell the most Fanny Farmer Chocolates. Trudging through the snow in the bitter Minnesota winters, we made our way up and down the streets of Minneapolis, hawking boxes of chocolates to anyone who'd stop and listen. We pitched the need to send two poor kids from the Northside of Minneapolis to camp. By selling those long, thin boxes of White Almond Bark, Assorted Chocolates, and Butter Creams, we earned enough money to pay the fees for two weeks of camp.

Once at camp, we learned about tying knots, archery, riflery, boating, canoeing, horseback riding, handling a knife and axe, plus a host of other abilities. Mastery of these skills marked an elite group of campers.

Camp Voyager sat next to Clear Lake. Four other lakes☐Fox Lake, Shoemaker Lake, Mud Lake, and Twin Lake—dotted the lush woods surrounding those waters. Shoemaker Lake sat furthest from the camp and was off-limits. But that didn't stop us. Any boy worth their salt hiked to the forbidden pond and back. A series of trodden paths connected all five lakes. Throughout the paths stood wooden signs. Counselors and camp leaders referred to them as 'guideposts.' The term was common in that day, although rarely used today. Yet, those guideposts became an essential part of our wilderness training.

The Camp Director—John—often said, "Following the guideposts is an important part of survival skills. Learning to follow instructions can mean the difference between enjoying out there," as he looked towards a dense, thickly wooded area, "Or getting lost." He pointed his finger to the first guidepost, which read, "Are you listening? The signs around camp will give you good pointers to help you enjoy camp, ensure you're safe, and give tips for living."

The guideposts were small wooden handmade signs fastened to posts lodged in the ground alongside those many paths. They kept us aware of our location, direction, and destination. Sometimes, they alerted us to danger, "Caution, Poison Oak." Or, "Beware, drop off." My favorite was, "Be on the lookout for bears." Like, if we came across a bear, what would we do?

Then there were the fable signs, "Quiet, no noise. Rip Van Winkle lives here." Remember Rip? The story of a frontier villager in colonial America who drinks their moonshine after meeting some shadowy pioneer Dutchmen and falls asleep in the Catskill Mountains only to awake twenty years later.

Another that I still remember fifty years later: "The wolf that ate Little Red Riding Hood lives here." Yeah, right?

The most critical guideposts were down at Clear Lake. Three paths intersected on the tiny little, muddy beach. There, guideposts ensured the safety of campers taking part in water activities. The most vital guidepost read, *"Find a buddy before entering the water."*

The buddy system—well-rehearsed and drilled repeatedly—is a system where each camper is responsible for looking out for another camper in the swimming area. It also helped lifeguards keep track of twenty campers at a time.

Assigning each swimmer with a number tag, two copper number tags dangling together from a hook on the Buddy Board represented one buddy team. Each buddy's responsibility was to monitor the other during the swim. Each swimmer's safety became the responsibility of the other buddy.

Every fifteen minutes, the lifeguard blew the whistle and called out, The lifeguard blew the whistle every fifteen minutes and called out, "Buddy Check!" Then the buddy-board attendant yelled, "Number one!" That pair of swimming buddies raised their hands together in response. Then, onto the next buddy pairing, "Number two!"

During my four summers up at Willow River as a camper and three more summers as a staff member, we never lost a single camper in those chilly waters in Northern Minnesota.

Back on the path, another signpost read, *"Your next step may be your itchiest."* We didn't pay attention to that guidepost. We ventured off the path into the thick, plush forest one day. Shortly after our return, the itching started. Then hives followed, too. We broke out with rashes of itchy, puffy, runny sores from head to toe. One camper ended up in the hospital with Poison Oak growing in every orifice of his miserable body. "Did you follow the guidepost?" A counselor asked. The answer was stupidly obvious.

We never got lost if we stayed on the path and followed the guideposts. Yet every year, some camper left the path, forsook a guidepost, preferring to hike through the thick growth unaccompanied. That affected everyone as the camp went into lockdown, canceling all activities until they found the camper. The discovered wanderer then faced sixty unhappy campers required to sit in their cabins all day waiting for the prodigal's return.

The guidepost at Mud Lake read, "Do not enter or swim in this lake; leeches." Well, a few leeches never kept anyone from swimming! An hour later, I stood with three other campers covered with the blood-sucking varmints. In a panic, we made the twenty-five-minute hike back to camp. Our counselor poured salt on the leeches. As they swiveled up, they fell off.

"Where was the adult supervision?" you might ask. It was a different day way back in the early 1970s. Kids roamed freely without the fears of today. Those guideposts helped ensure our safety, although campers often learned lessons the hard way. That was part of the experience.

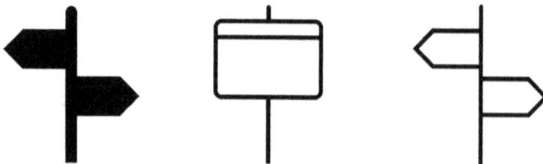

Guideposts

In this book, I offer mental health guideposts for your consideration. They come from decades of interacting with missionaries, pastors, and other Christians and in learning to deal with my own mental health.

Please understand that I am not a professional health worker, therapist, psychologist, or psychiatrist.

But I'm learning to live by the Scripture,

That's why **I take pleasure** in *my weaknesses*, and in the insults, hardships, persecutions, and troubles that I suffer for Christ. For when I am weak, then I am strong.

2 Corinthians 12:10 Emphasis Mine

Now, I'm not anywhere as spiritual as the Apostle Paul. Anger, despair, puzzlement, and loss face off with me daily. Some days, there's victory. Other days begin in a mental dungeon.

I'm reminded from the Bible that hope and strength are available, even in severe weakness. Weakness can point us toward God as we allow him to become our sanctuary and strength. In weakness, we can move forward.

I've learned never to say never with mental health. I've witnessed too many of God's people succumb to mental maladies, believing their faith should put them above such afflictions. These often become the castaways of the Church.

This book is divided into four parts:

Part One: Christian Mental Health Misnomers
Part Two: Lifting Mental Health Stigmas
Part Three: Warning Signs
Part Four: Positive Mental Health Practices

Part 1

Christian Mental Health Misnomers

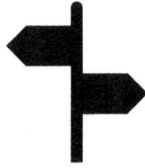

Guidepost #1

Never Say Never

Say It Ain't So!

I DIDN'T WANT TO GET out of bed on a particular Monday in Uganda. I wanted to throw a shoe at that rooster's head. I wondered if people would notice if the metal workshop worker clanging across the street suddenly went missing.

I didn't want to wage war with the mice in my kitchen anymore. I just wanted to stay indoors with the fan running longer. I didn't want to face the heat or the endless sea of haunted faces I knew were probably waiting for me at the office. It felt like the stark winter landscape, snow blanketing the spindling trees, everything dry and bare.

Depression is a winter of the soul. Everything muted.

I felt bad, and I felt guilty for feeling bad. What would people think of me if they knew there were days to even weeks when I felt depressed? [2]

You've just met Sarita. A real person. A real missionary. An individual struggling with mental health. Let me introduce you to some others.

David

I lived in Asia for over 25 years. Much of that time, I struggled with mental health concerns. I still have mental health issues. I cringe as I write that: "mental health issues." It seems like a lot of language surrounding mental health perpetuates negative stereotypes. But I'd rather say I have "issues" than say I still have mental health problems or a mental illness.[3]

Valarie

As I lay face down on the cold, hard floor of our apartment in El Salvador, a man held a gun to the back of my head as his three companions took away our meager possessions.

Thankfully, the babies stayed asleep despite the clothes thrown upon them as the robbers looked for treasure. The three informed the last man to "take care" of us.

However, as he left, he whispered, "It is only because of your God," and shut the door.

This story describes one of many traumatic events DeLonn and I faced during our 29-year missionary career, yet we never once thought of leaving the field.[4]

Katie

I experienced my first (and worst) season of depression the year after graduating university. I went on a missions internship to Papua New Guinea and endured two months of vicious team conflict, food poisoning, kidney stones, you name it, I probably had it.

For the following six months, I was very sick from an undiagnosed illness that turned out to be recurring malaria. A hard relationship break-up sent me spiraling into a season of depression for about two years.

Since recovering from that dark period, I've experienced depression several times while serving on the mission field. Close team members also struggled with anxiety and depression. At times, I've felt like I'm treading water, holding my head above the waves.

If that's you, painting on the happy Christian face, trying to serve God while loving people, trying to make it through the day - I understand. I've been there. And you're not alone. [5]

Agoraphobic Missionary

Sitting in my office in Northern Minnesota, my administrative assistant informed me of a phone call, "Pastor, sorry to bother you, but I think you need to take this call right now."

I answered, "Hello, this is pastor Don."

A sobbing missionary began.

"Hello, this is R_____ M_____. Your church supports us. I'm sorry to inform you we can't return to Ukraine. We are in Iowa right now. We won't be able to return to the field."

A further conversation revealed his wife suffered from severe agoraphobia. This is an overwhelming fear of leaving the home.[6] After receiving a year of treatment, she still couldn't leave their rented house.

'Spiritual leaders' surrounding them credited her affliction to 'spiritual warfare,' a 'lack of faith,' or a 'failure of obedience.' Biblical counselors at their church concluded the missionary wife's problem was because of some hidden sin or a failure to trust God.

Without compensation, care, or preparation, their agency ended their missionary employment. The missionary—a MK or missionary kid—lost the only life he'd ever known.

R_____ shared with me, "It's like I'm a refugee here in Iowa. I hate it, but I don't know what else to do. And our mission agency abandoned us."

With that—like so many others—their sending church dropped all financial support. He stood unemployed without insurance to care for his wife.

After listening to that missionary for over an hour, I offered these words.

"R_____, thank you for your faithful years of service. Thanks for putting your wife's needs above your desire for ministry and missionary life.

Don't allow the title of 'missionary' to define who you are. You and your wife are children of God. Beloved in every way.

Find someone who can help your wife. A specialist with skills to deal with your wife's condition. Someone who understands missionaries and the stressful lives they live. Believe it or not, your wife is not the only agoraphobic I know within missionary ranks and among pastors, too.

God is faithful. May he show you purpose in all of this. You're not a failure. You are my hero. God will right this one day."

With that, the church I pastored sent the abandoned missionary couple a generous gift to help them through their financial difficulties.

Does any of this surprise you? Happens all the time.

Jean

Several years ago, while speaking at a missionary retreat in Central America, a missionary couple asked to talk to Kathy and me. Sitting in front of the small lecture hall, the husband began, "We've got a big problem." After rambling for about thirty minutes, I asked, "What's your big problem?"

He blurted out, "Oh, yes! We've a big problem. Our daughter, Jane—not her real name—is cutting. We just found out the other day."

I replied, "I'm so very sorry about this. May I ask you a few questions to gain some understanding of your situation?" To this, he agreed, and we began.

"When did Jean start cutting?"

"I don't know."

"What part of her body is she cutting?"

"Well, her arms, but I don't know if she's cutting anywhere else."

"How is she cutting herself?"

"I don't know. What do you mean?"

"Is she cutting herself up and down or from side to side? Across the wrist or up the arm?"

"I'm not sure."

That small conversation told me volumes. Dad was not engaged in his daughter's life.
Mom's silence seemed imposed. Wanting to speak up, a glance from the husband silenced her.

I asked, "What's going on here?" nodding in both directions towards each one.

Flood gates of emotions opened.

Mom blurted out, "We don't know who to talk to. It's not like anyone really cares about us way out here. We don't even know the new pastor of our sending church. And I don't want everyone in the church to know about this."

Dad commandeered the conversation again, exclaiming, "We could lose all our support if anyone finds out."

He went on about the possibility of their mission agency firing them, their sending church dropping their backing, and a host of other concerns.

What I heard little about was Jean.

I raised my arms straight out in front of me with my hands pointing forward towards them with palms facing down. Then I asked, "If my right hand is your ministry, and my left hand is your daughter, help me understand." With that, I began lowering my right hand, saying, "So… you're worried about losing your ministry," then raising my right hand back to its original position, I began dropping my left hand, "Or you're worried about losing your daughter."

Which is most important to you?

From then on, we talked about Jean. After two more sessions, the couple acted. You know what happened?

Upon hearing their report, the new pastor of their sending church asked, "What can we do to help?" Their mission agency introduced them to a female therapist specializing in MK and TCK teenage women. She was a single missionary, and she began cutting under the intense stress of single missionary life. Hiding the secret for as long as possible, she reached out for help.

She enrolled at Liberty University after two years of therapy and biblical counseling. Earning her PhD in counseling, she purposed to help as many missionary women as possible.

Way Back in 84

It was 1984, and we were young rookie missionaries attending the first of dozens of mission conferences. The speaker that night was a veteran missionary serving in South America. Back in those days, he shared his slide presentation. What was missing in the presentation was his wife. Then he told the story.

During their twelfth year of missionary work, his wife suffered bouts of depression. Afraid, they told no one. Her condition continued to deteriorate. One day, after returning from a meeting with national pastors, he called out to his wife. She didn't answer.

He found her body in a back room. She'd taken her life. As he spoke of the tragedy, words rang out that I can still remember almost forty years later.

"I didn't know what to do… about my wife's depression. Now she's gone."

That heartbreak unfolded as the missionary talked about how friends distanced themselves. Many churches dropped his financial support. The mission agency he served under, having a policy of not allowing single males to serve, dismissed him, too.

Does any of this surprise you?

There he stood, bereft of companionship and financial viability. I didn't quite know what to make of it all. Young and excited about our own missionary calling, Kathy and I soon forgot about that night, and the grieving cross-cultural worker.

I'd like to tell you it's the only missionary suicide I know of, but regrettably, after a bit of pondering, four missionaries come to mind from past decades who ended their own lives, and two pastors as well. Just last week, I attended the funeral of a young pastor who ended his life after a long struggle with depression.

Jamie

Dear Depression,

We've known each other for quite some time now. The first time I met you, I never got your name. You extended a hand like you were some kind of savior, arrived to shield me from the dark side of life.

Your quiet demeanor enamored me. I assumed maybe you knew something I didn't. I was quite sick, isolated by my pain and fears, and had no labels for the physical distress I was experiencing.

Now I have the courage to tell you the truth: you are a terrible friend. You come calling when I least expect it, and honestly, I don't appreciate it. I open the door, expecting help, or an amazon package, and instead, it's you. You tell me what I can't do, laying across my path like an inconvenient truth, but the reality is you are just inconvenient.

I won't be answering your calls or opening the door anymore. I have a new friend. Well really, we've been talking the whole time. For all the times you put glue on my pillow and rubbed my face in my failures, he brought me donuts, called me beloved, and organized my closet (like only the savior of the world can). It's crazy; we can talk for hours about anything, and he just looks at me like there is nowhere else in the world he would rather be. It's pretty sweet.

Yeah, I'm sticking with him.[7]

Tina

Tina was the wife of a retired pastor in Waukesha, Wisconsin. I met her while accompanying my son to purchase a puppy.

While talking, she asked about my occupation. Mentioning the years of my missionary experience and then pastoring a church, she replied,

"I can never walk into church again. Just entering makes me ill."

Stacy

Stacy, also the wife of a retired pastor, stayed confined to her home. She ventured out only for medical treatment. Having served in the same church for over thirty years, she shared, "That church used us up."

Stacy and her husband receive few visitors, living as hermits.

Thomas

Thomas is probably the most talented person I've ever known. After the tragic death of a foster child in their home from S.I.D.S., he and his wife suffered immense mental anguish.

Six months later, still numb from the experience, their senior pastor launched into him, "It's not like she was your daughter. She was a foster child. Get it together."

With that, Thomas followed Jesus right out the door of the church, never to return. He and his wife never fully recovered from that terrible day, or the lack of compassion from those claiming to love them.

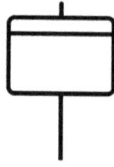

Reflection

Can you identify with any of these people?

How would you try to help someone in a similar situation?

What about your own mental health these days?

Mental health affects Christians, too. ?????

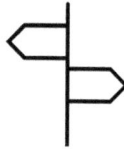

Making the Case for Mental Health

Here's the thing. Overwhelming evidence in the Bible shows God cares about our mental health.

The Bible is full of people struggling with their mental health.

There's a discouraged and afraid Elijah, asking God to end his life.

Jonah sitting under a tree, wishing himself dead.

Hannah crying because of her barren state, begging for a child.

23

King David, at the end of his rope, in deep despair.

Moses asking God to kill him.

Jeremiah wrestling with loneliness and insecurity.

Job losing everything.

Even Jesus deeply anguished in the Garden.

These are only a few examples in Scripture. God led these mentally anguished people towards emotional and mental health.

From the context of Scripture, we see that many in the Bible struggled with mental health. Now, let's discover the degree to which God cares and delve into God's mental health perspective.

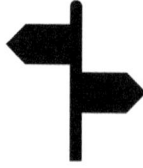

Guidepost #2

God Cares About Mental Health

A CHRISTIAN MISCONCEPTION EXISTS THAT faith and mental illness can't coexist apart from sin or lack of trust in God.

A well-meaning Christian leader shot back at me the other day, "Faith is the answer to mental illness. Those who live by faith don't struggle with their mental health. It they do, it's because they're out of God's will."

If that is true, then countless Christians are outside of the 'will of God,' including myself. And what about those people in the Bible who wrestled with their mental health? Only by spiritualizing their accounts can you dismiss the obvious.

The opposite is true. Faith doesn't guarantee a life unhindered by mental illness.

Many common ailments associated with mental health creep upon missionaries, pastors, and other Christians. Within our churches sit hosts of people besieged with poor mental health: anxiety, panic attacks, and depression are just a few.[8] The demands placed on clergy, pastors, and missionaries put them at far greater risk of depression than their church congregants. [9] Looking for hope, faithful people trying to live a Christian life wake up many mornings in mental despair.

What does the Bible say about this?

The Bible doesn't explicitly refer to 'mental health' in the manner we use the term today. However, Scripture talks about our emotions, mind, soul, and heart. In this, the Bible alludes to mental health often.

Depressed People in the Bible

The Old Testament contains many examples of notable people who struggled with depression:

Job the Wealthy Farmer:

> Why wasn't I born dead? Why didn't I die as I came from the womb?.... I have no peace, no quietness. I have no rest; only trouble comes.
>
> Job 3:11, 26

Moses the Meek Leader:

> I am not able to bear all these people alone. The burden is too heavy for me. If You treat me like this, please kill me here and now if I have found favor in Your sight and do not let me see my wretchedness!
>
> Numbers 11:14-17 NKJV

Hannah the Barren Mother:

> 'Oh no, sir!' she replied. 'I haven't been drinking wine or anything stronger. But I am very discouraged, and I was pouring out my heart to the Lord. Don't think I am a wicked woman! For I have been praying out of great anguish and sorrow.'
>
> 1 Samuel 1:15-16

Elijah the Often Mentally Ill Ignored Prophet:

'I have had enough, Lord,' he said. 'Take my life, for I am no better than my ancestors who have already died.'

1 Kings 19:4

King David the Giant Slayer:

How long must I struggle with anguish in my soul, with sorrow in my heart every day? I am dying from grief; my years are shortened by sadness. Sin has drained my strength; I am wasting away from within.

Psalm 13:2; 31:10

Heman the Son of Korah:

I am forgotten, cut off from your care. You have thrown me into the lowest pit, into the darkest depths. Your anger weighs me down; with wave after wave you have engulfed me.

Psalm 88:5-7

Jonah the Reluctant Missionary:

Just kill me now, Lord! I'd rather be dead than alive if what I predicted will not happen.

Jonah 4:3

Jeremiah the Weeper:

I have cried until the tears no longer come; my heart is broken.

Lamentations 2:11

Paul the Apostle:

> We think you ought to know, dear brothers and sisters, about the trouble we went through in the province of Asia. We were crushed and overwhelmed beyond our ability to endure, and we thought we would never live through it.
>
> 2 Corinthians 1:8

It's interesting to note that of these nine people listed from the Bible, four—Job, Moses, Elijah, and Jonah—all displayed intense suicidal ideations. We tend to over-spiritualize these dialogues, failing to see these God-followers as those who contemplated ending their lives.

The Bible and Mental Health

Anxiety has been a continuous challenge for generations. King Solomon acknowledged this 3,000 years ago:

"Anxiety weighs down the heart…" Proverbs 12:25 NIV

The Gesenius Hebrew-Chaldee Lexicon defines 'anxiety' as "Fear, dread, and anxious care." We find the same Hebrew word in Jeremiah 49:23, describing anxiety as agitated waves of the sea or ocean.[10]

Agitated waves. Fearful, anxious living.

A continuous churning up of worries, concerns, and trepidation within our hearts and minds.

The Apostle Paul desired for his friends at the church in Corinth: "I want you to be free from anxieties…" I Corinthians 7:32 ESV

God cares about our mental health. It's mentioned too many times in Scripture to ignore.

28

A Decisive Answer for Depression:

But <u>as a result</u>, we *stopped relying on ourselves* and [learned to rely only on God,] who raises the dead.

2 Corinthians 1:9 Emphasis Mine

Ultimately, regardless of the treatment I'm receiving for my PTSD and depression, this is the goal. I set this before myself daily, trusting God as I take my meds for hypertension, heart, and PTSD. As my body wastes away with Muscular Dystrophy, and my mind replays the harsh events of growing up in Minnesota along with my memories of the killing fields in Africa, trusting God brings me complete peace. God is my peace.

One day, God will make everything right according to his plans and purpose. Romans 8:28

I understand that the 'everything' in this verse is not always now. God causes everything to work out for 'good,' but the verse doesn't promise 'good' fulfillment in our timelines. This good is eternity's good, God's plan for the ages, and how it fits into his purpose. That is where I put my hope. That one day, God will right all this.

He will *wipe every tear* from their eyes, and there will be no more death or sorrow or crying or pain. All these things are gone forever.

Revelation 21:4

It's in this that God cares for us. The old hymn says, "*There's a land that is fairer than this*; in the sweet by and by, we shall meet on that beautiful shore." The problem is that we live in the troubled here and now.

God cares about your mental health.

Knowing that God wants us to live meaningful lives, even in physical and mental health challenges,

29

keeps me going. Knowing that God wants us to live meaningful lives, even with physical and mental health challenges, keeps me going. The Bible recognizes that life is challenging but also promises that God is a faithful companion, "He will never leave us nor forsake us." Hebrews 13:5

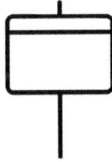

Reflection

What were your thoughts about mental health before reading this chapter?

How about now?

What about your own mental health?

Suggested Resources to Improve Your Mental Health

Winning the War in Your Mind: Change Your Thinking, Change Your Life by Craig Groeschel.

Your Brain Is Always Listening: Tame the Hidden Dragons That Control Your Happiness, Habits, and Hang-Ups by Daniel G. Amen.

Out of the Cave: Stepping into the Light when Depression Darkens What You See by Chris Hodges.

Get Out of Your Head: Stopping the Spiral of Toxic Thoughts By Jennie Allen.

Telling Yourself the Truth: Find Your Way Out of Depression, Anxiety, Fear, Anger, and Other Common Problems by Applying the Principles of Misbelief Therapy by William Backus and Marie Chapian.

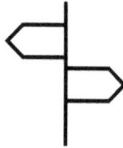

Making the Case

One major hurdle with pastors and missionaries is the notion of mental illness invincibility.

"That can never happen to me. It must never happen to me."

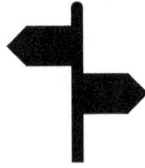

Guidepost #3

Christian Mental Health Invincibility is a Myth

WITHIN CHRISTIAN RANKS, THERE OFTEN exists a brash attitude of Christian invincibility towards mental health ailments.

It can't happen to me because I'm a dedicated Christian.

A Scripture often leaned upon in this interpretation is 2 Timothy 1:7, when Paul encouraged the young Timothy:

For God hath not given us the spirit of fear; but of power, and of love, and of a sound mind. KJV

A close look at this verse shows it doesn't speak to mental health but to learning the art of self-discipline.

From where does this mental health invincibility myth come? Why is this mentality so prevalent in some Christian circles? A philosophy called the Just-world hypothesis is pervasive in our churches today. It holds:

That the world is fair, and consequently, that the moral standings of our actions will determine our outcomes. This viewpoint causes us to believe that those who do good will be rewarded, and those who exhibit negative behaviors will be punished. [11]

This thinking breeds patterns like, "If I'm focused upon God and the Bible, my reward is prosperous, even mental health." Some might call this. However, if I struggle with depression, for example, that's the result of some sin in my life for which God punishes me. As one explosive man leaned into me, erupting, "Those who walk close to God never get depressed."

Really?

There's a juxtaposition of belief here in the Church. On the one hand, God forgives us for our wrongdoings. God's grace through his son delivers us from the consequences of sin, securing eternal life for us. Thank goodness. However, in daily Christian living, we often drift away from grace. We believe that through the strength of our faith, we secure God's favor. This favor keeps us from suffering, sickness, and mental illness. Our faith becomes our faith. What I believe makes it so because I think it is so.

By our faith, 'we get what we deserve.'
Good faith, excellent results.
Poor faith, poor results.
Bad faith, meh, you get what you believe.

Acknowledging your mental health needs must become a priority.

Many cling to an old saying, "God will never give you more than you can handle."

The problem with that statement is it's not true. Not even close. How does faith develop and mature if God gives me only what I can handle for myself? God often allows obstacles beyond our abilities, forcing us to trust him. Faith is all about gaining the ability to overcome by trusting in God's ability. James 1:5-6

I think that *hosts of people sitting in the Church place their faith in their faith.* How a person believes determines the good or bad treatment God allows in their life. If you're close to God, God is near you, rewarding you with health and opulence.

As a lady recently drawled at me in church, "People__ who__ are__ close__ to__ God__ don't__ have__ PTSD!"

My response was, "Have you ever read the Bible?"

Read the famous eleventh chapter of Hebrews called the Faith Chapter. Look at what happened to those faith-filled people at the end of that chapter.

What about Elijah, Job, Jonah, or Joseph? Or even King David, a Man After God's Own Heart? He experienced immense mental anguish. Marriage problems, incest, family murders, betrayals, ill health, and, in the early days, a king who continuously tried to murder him. Then, in his golden years, David's son led an uprising. Stealing his kingship, Absalom raped many of David's wives. Only by killing his son did he regain the throne. In David's psalms, you'll often find a depressed king trying to make life work. A faith-filled believer, yet depressed.

There are no guarantees we get through this life unafflicted by mental health issues. Not even for Christians. The sooner we understand this, the more diligent we can become in guarding our own mental health.

Where do my Christian friends suffering from Bipolar Disorder turn to for help under such teaching? Many are told there's no such thing as Bipolar Disorder. The Bible doesn't make allowances for such things. Really? Ever study King Saul's life?

Yesterday, on the phone with a pastor friend, also suffering from FSHD Muscular Dystrophy, we discussed the emotional component of living with this long-term disabling disease. He shared:

"Don, recently, another pastor said, 'If you had enough faith, you'd not be struggling with your disease.' That angered me."

That's a savagely ignorant person. This kind of shallowness leaves little place for mental struggles to find empathy and belonging within the Church. Perhaps that's a reason so many mental strugglers leave the Church.

Then he also added, "My son shared with me that a pastor friend of his doesn't believe in such a thing as 'mental illness.' I told him to stay as far away from that guy as possible."

I doubt many contemplate mental health when preparing for church employment. It wasn't until fairly recently that missionary organizations began looking at their candidates' emotional well-being before approving them for service. It's interesting that when I joined a paid on-call fire department, they required me to undergo a psychological examination. Yet, during my interviews for the lead pastor, both churches that hired me never required a psychological profile.

If spiritual leaders are to shepherd their congregations well, we must weigh together both mental and spiritual health. Looking back, I now realize that accepting the pastorate while struggling with severe PTSD was both unhealthy and unwise. But, I didn't know the degree of my mental frailty. A psychological profile would have uncovered my condition and need for help.

The Messed-Up Missionary

During my many years in South Africa, I often frequented Wimpy's. Seemed like every town in South Africa sported a Wimpy's in those days. It was a hamburger joint that was so much more than just a fast-food establishment.

There, you enjoyed table service with your food served on glass plates with real cutlery, not plastic forks and knives. Why plates and silverware for hamburgers and french fries? That's the unique nature of life in many Wimpy's. Many South Africans eat their burgers and chips—french fries—with a knife and fork. It's considered appropriate for dining.

Our favorite reason for visiting was their coffee. Many mornings took place at Wimpy's over a beautiful cup of hot steaming coffee with whipped hot milk and a shovel full of sugar. Many missionary meetings occurred at Wimpy's throughout Southern Africa as well. Wimpy's is where I met another missionary named Ian, who was up in Botswana.

Ian was a single British missionary who lived in a mud hut among the Kalanga people. My son Daniel and I drove hundreds of miles out of South Africa up into Botswana to meet with him.

What started out as a casual conversation turned into a thought-provoking misfortune. Ian shared his setbacks and discouragements in Botswana. Under supported, he struggled to provide for himself, let alone build a ministry. There were glimmers of success, too. Earlier, he took us to a little shoemaking shop. After that, to a group of weavers who produced and sold their African rugs and then to a leather shop. He taught Kalanga people how to start and run successful businesses. A small, thriving community existed because of Ian.

Ian impressed me, but he showed all the signs of severe depression. He longed for a soulmate, having just celebrated his thirty-first birthday with no hope of meeting a missionary woman who might endure the harsh surroundings of missionary life.

Then, his talk turned dark. "Most mornings, I can hardly get out of bed now. There is no strength or willpower. I mean, what am I here for, anyway?"

I raised my shoulders as if to say, "I don't know."

Then he continued. "There is no one out here like me to talk with. I've considered returning to England but don't even have the money to buy a ticket." Then he slumped, "I'm just faffing around here, anyway. I feel so smarmy."

I smiled, not really understanding what he meant by that last expression. Then he looked at me.

36

"You know, I could just walk deep into the bush some night and never come back. No one would miss me."

Ian was in trouble. He sensed it but didn't know the degree to which his mental health deteriorated. When suicidal ideation presents itself, a person is in distress. He ended with, "I'm pretty messed up."

I encouraged him to take a furlough. Find the money. Ask for it. Beg for it. Return to England. It'd been ten years since he'd seen his family.

He took my advice. Returned to England. Got a physical. Discovered he suffered from hyperthyroidism, and while undergoing chemotherapy, met a lovely Irish lass and got married. Last I heard, he still returned to Botswana regularly to encourage his Kalanga friends.

Recently, a friend shared with me a troubling development in his life. Conner was always a successful, positive individual. It surprised him that after suffering from Covid-19, he began struggling with deep bouts of depression.

"It's never happened to me before; depression. But ever since Covid, I've struggled with it. I'm getting help from my doctor, and my pastor understands such things. He's helped me a lot. But it's tough to deal with."

Never say mental health decline can't happen to you. Be aware. Mental health deterioration can happen to anyone, even a missionary or pastor. Even you. It's befallen many Christ-followers. Be mindful of your mental health condition.

Christian Mental Health Taboos

There's long been a misconception in the Church, especially among Evangelical Christians, that somehow mental illness results from spiritual incompetence. That response has done more damage than good.

The Church's response?

Mental illness is a sign of weakness. Chin up! Toughen up! Get it together, man! In my case with PTSD, one pastor launched into me, "There's no such thing! You've bought into a lie! You're self-victimizing yourself![12] Ministry is tough everywhere. Stop being a wuss."

No medications; just surrender your mental illness to God. What about individuals who suffer from migraines? Do they take Tylenol for their headaches? Of course, they do. "Why don't they just surrender their migraines to God?"

Almost daily, I surrender my PTSD to God, asking for strength, humility, and self-control. Often, my prayer goes, "God, please give me a mentally peaceful day." Then, I take my medication.

Here's the thing, rarely can mental illness be prayed away,[13] no more than you can prevent death's ultimate condition. These frail bodies suffer sickness and eventually die. No one has beat those odds. Well, there is Elijah and Melchizedek, but that's another discussion altogether. Because of Adam's sin, our frail, dying persons must undergo the transformation of death, bridging this life to the next.

This is just God's way of testing you. I like what Rev. Alba Onofrio—spiritual strategist at Soulforce—has to say about this idea:

> I don't believe God gives us mental illness or cancer or any other suffering as a test of our faith or a punishment for the lack thereof. And I know from the incredibly high statistics of suicide among certain marginalized communities that sometimes we are absolutely faced with more than we have tools to handle.[14]

I can tell you from the few pastors and missionaries I've known who've taken their lives that Alba's words appear very accurate. I know that before receiving professional help, an overwhelming sense of doom almost finished me.

God must be punishing you for some sin in your life. I remember when my son Dan was in intensive care at Children's Hospital in Dallas, Texas. A well-meaning, although incredibly insensitive, member of the church arrived. The first words from her mouth were, "Is there some sin we can pray with you about?"

Tersely, I replied, "Yes, let's pray that you will leave."

I get grumpy at times.

Your faith is weak. Really? Because of PTSD, Bipolar disorder, depression, or some other mental illness? Really? Is mental illness a mark of weak faith? I think the opposite is true. People with mental illnesses who still focus their trust in God are faith champions of the Church.

Try launching out of bed in a cold sweat some night, reliving a scene of seeing children being murdered during your missionary years of service. Then say, "God, I will learn to trust you in all this."

Weak faith? Quite the opposite.

Want to know why so many missionaries leave the faith upon leaving their fields of service? Try being a missionary in a third-world country. Get out with the people. Live in their lifestyles. You'll soon find out.

Or many pastors who, upon leaving their pastorates, leave the Church, too. American pastors are among the most stressed-out people I've ever known. And there's just reason for their stress. American congregations present one of the strongest challenges to anyone's sanity because of the incredible, sometimes impossible, demands placed upon their clergy.

That's why Christians—including pastors and missionaries—disappear from the church. Plus, the shame and despair they live with, believing themselves spiritually impotent because of their mental health woes.

What Can We Do?

Offer a Ministry of Presence. Don't try to fix a person who struggles with a mental ailment. Instead, offer a listening ear, a kind and well-placed honest word.

Like, "I don't understand what you're going through, but I'm here for you." Then, be there.

Lead Pastor of Sojourn Community Church's Midtown campus in Louisville, Kentucky, says, 'Being present means being on call to serve.' Sometimes, just being with someone and giving undivided attention and witnessing is the best thing to offer.[15]

Still unconvinced?

Famous Messed-Up Christian Leaders

A. B. Simpson, founder of the Christian and Missionary Alliance: "I fell into the slough of despondency so deep that… work was impossible… I wandered about deeply depressed. All things in life looked dark and withered."

Adoniram Judson, missionary to Burma: "God is to me the Great Unknown. I believe in him, but I find him not."

David Brainerd, missionary to native Americans, "I live in the most lonely melancholy desert… My soul was weary of life. I longed for death, beyond measure." [16]

Mary Morrison, her husband Robert Morrison (China), wrote, "My poor afflicted Mary… She walks in darkness and has no light." [17]

Charles Haddon Spurgeon, the famed English preacher of the 19th century, battled depression his entire ministry. In one of his sermons, he said:

> You may surround yourself with all the comforts of life and yet be in wretchedness more gloomy than death if the spirits are depressed. You may have no outward cause whatever for sorrow and yet if the mind is dejected, the brightest sunshine will not relieve your gloom.

> … There are times when all our evidences get clouded, and all our joys are fled. Though we may still cling to the Cross, *yet it is with a desperate grasp.*[18] Emphasis mine.

"Yet it is with a desperate grasp." A very accurate descriptor of my PTSD battle over the years.

Hannah Allen was a nonconformist writer in England during the 17th century. While not a significant influence in church history like Charles Wesley or Martin Luther, she was an everyday Christian who wrote about her 'religious melancholy' as it was called in that day. In her *Journals of Affliction* she writes:

> Lord, I know not what to do, only mine eyes are up to thee, the Devil still keeps me under dreadful bondage, and in sad distress and wo[e]… [19]

Martin Luther the Father of the Reformation once wrote his good friend:

> I almost lost Christ in the waves of blast and despair and blasphemy against God, but God was moved by the prayers of the saints and began to take pity on me and rescued my soul from the lowest hell. [20]

Never say you'll never face a mental health crisis. Pastor, don't believe you're beyond such afflictions. Christian, don't think that your religious service and piety exempt you from mental frailties. Satan, our adversary, seeks to take us out of the race. This fallen angelic being strikes, mental health being one effective weapon against God's people.

Care for your mental health as you do your physical self.

Be on guard.

Be aware.

Pay attention to what you view.

Watch how you think.

Listen to the conversations in your head. Ask yourself, "Are my thoughts accurate and healthy?"

Prayer alone rarely eliminates mental illnesses.

Most of all, if you need help, please get help.

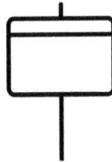

Mental Health Self-Assessment

How's your emotional condition these days?

Excellent, good, ok, meh, poor, or....?

Talk with your spouse, colleague, or friend. How are you doing? Really...

Do they agree with your evaluation of yourself?

Do you agree with theirs?

Are you grumpy?

Tired and worn out?

A Ministry of Presence is a call to silent service.

42

In the dumps?

Feeling hopeless, "What's the point of it all?"

Additional Resources for Consideration

Christians Get Depressed Too: Hope and Help for Depressed People by David P Murray. Available on Amazon.

I highly recommend reading *Companions in the Darkness: Seven Saints Who Struggled With Depression* by Diana Gruver.

> The church's relationship with depression has been fraught: for centuries, depression was assumed to be evidence of personal sin or even demonic influence… In recent years the conversation has begun to change, and the stigma has lessened—but as anyone who suffers from depression knows, we still have a long way to go.
>
> Diana Gruver

Part II

Lifting Mental Health Stigmas

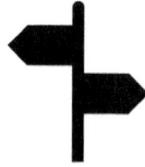

Guidepost #4

Admit When You Need Help

That Day

SITTING IN THE WAITING ROOM that day at Arden Hills Psychological Services, the thought of leaving circled my mind. I didn't belong there. I wasn't like those sitting around me. They needed a Christian shrink; I did not.

Everything about me screamed inside, "THIS IS NOT FOR ME!" The biblical counseling training received under well-meaning, knowledgeable counselors railed against anything with the word 'psychology' in it. But... even though I prayed it through, memorized the Scriptures, attempted to trust God, and followed a host of other spiritual prescriptions, my condition deteriorated.

The sleepless nights, noise aversion—any noise—the cold sweats, nightmares, and extremes in temperaments pushed me towards seeing a pastor friend who'd reached out to me. He sensed that something wasn't right in my well-being. Randy pastored a large Evangelical Free church in the Twin Cities, Minnesota. Sharing the darkness in my life, Randy smiled and said, "That's alright, Don. We'll get some answers for you." The sleepless nights, aversion to noise—any noise—the cold sweats, nightmares, and extremes in temperaments pushed me towards seeing a pastor friend who'd reached out to me. He sensed that something wasn't right in my wellbeing. Randy pastored a large Evangelical Free church in the Twin Cities, Minnesota. Sharing the darkness in my life, Randy smiled and said, "That's alright Don. We'll get some answers for you."

With that, he gave me the number of a Christian therapist to call and added, "Don't worry about paying for it. Our church will cover the costs." This relieved me of one stressor: the church I pastored offered no medical insurance coverage.

That day, sitting in the waiting room, knowing I needed help, my soul wanted to hide. "Anywhere but here," I thought. Yet my mind also whispered, "You need help. You know you do." I argued with myself,

You are a Christian!

A missionary!

Now, a pastor!

What will people think?

Come on! Shape up, Donald, you are better than this!

As I rose, making my way towards the exit, a small statured-man entered the lobby from a side door and called out, "Don."

That day, I met Tom. From a pastor's home, Tom studied at Bethel University and Rosemead School of Psychology, earning his credentials to become a highly sought-after therapist.

Tom immediately set me at ease with his calm demeanor and quiet voice. Once in his office, floodgates of emotion, puzzlement, and concerns poured out. That day, I did most of the talking. After ninety minutes of talking nonstop, I ended with, "Tom, what's wrong with me?"

Four sessions later came the diagnosis; PTSD.

My problem was not of spiritual causation. No willful sin, lack of faith, or failure led to my PTSD. This affliction came from traumatic images and experiences embedded in my brain both in my childhood and on the killing fields near the Zulu Kingdom in KwaZulu, Natal, South Africa.

Added to that was a blow to the head that sent me to a South African ER and into intensive care and six months of therapy trying to speak again without stuttering. What was diagnosed as a mild brain injury turned out to be not so mild, causing me undue complications from then on.

My son Daniel told me, "Dad, after your head injury, you changed." Dan was right.

I learned that PTSD was perhaps not as much of a mental illness of shame as a physical injury to my brain. Life changed that day I met Tom. In coping with the effects of my trauma, only then did hope emerge.

Trauma and the Brain

When trauma ruminates in the limbic system's amygdala, it closes the door on the brain's rational part—the prefrontal cortex—and replays a past event or events, as if they were taking place in real-time.

The trauma of holding a six-year-old Zulu girl dying of AIDS raped a few years earlier played itself repeatedly in my mind. The shock of witnessing people killed, murdered, or set on fire repeated live time in my brain.

Countless nights, I shot up out of bed drenched with sweat, grabbing my chest as if someone was stabbing me. Except, no one was there but me. Every violent dream carried a sense of entrapment, an impossible escape toward safety. Certain sounds still rip a hole through me.

This is PTSD.

While much larger, the prefrontal cortex often sits on the sidelines, failing to communicate with the smaller limbic system that a traumatic event is over. Until my brain received help to understand and deal with PTSD, nothing else helped. Reading the Scriptures, prayer, and spiritual disciplines did not address to the issue. However, in learning to empower my rational brain—prefrontal cortex—I gained control over my emotional brain, the limbic system.

My friends, can you pray away mental illness? Yes and no. I know that statement will rile some of you theologically.

A Lifeway Research Survey found that half of all evangelical, fundamental, born-again Christians believe prayer and Bible study alone can overcome a serious mental illness. Dr. Linda Mintle, in the survey, notes,

> God sees the whole picture. He knows what is best for us. Sometimes, the outcome of someone struggling with a mental illness is a closer walk for family members, even a conversion can happen as people depend on God. We don't know how God uses the brokenness of our lives.[21]

Dr. Mintle encourages, "I think we need to be careful in limiting God to heal the way we think he should." [22]

That Day

The term 'mental health' acquired a personal meaning that day. I suffered from a mental health condition, Post Traumatic Stress Disorder. A condition that much of my faith world ignores is ignorant of, fears, or denies its legitimacy.

In coping with the effects of trauma, only then did hope emerge.

A disorder that much of my faith-world ignores, is ignorant of, fears, or denies its legitimacy. That day, our recovery—Kathy's and mine—led us in a new direction. Understanding my problem allowed me to seek a solution-focused answer to what had ailed me for so long.

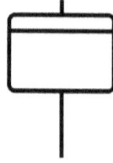

What about you?

How's your mental health?

Have you experienced a 'That Day?'

Who can you talk with about your 'That Day?'

Additional Resources for Consideration

To Hell, Back, and Beyond: A PTSD Journey, When Faith and Trauma Collide by Don Mingo

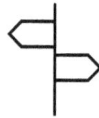

Where Do Mental Health Issues Come From?

Epigenetic inheritance—a parent's experience may be passed down to their children—appears linked to several disorders such as anxiety, stress, depression, schizophrenia, and addiction,[23] but many mental ailments may hinge upon a single or series of past traumatic events in which a person cognitively copes with poorly.

Mental Health often revolves around past events in our lives. Dealing with our past becomes a necessary step toward living in our present. Only then can we move forward in our futures.

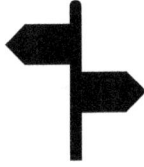

Guidepost #5

Learn to Deal With Your Past or it Will Deal With You

NO MATTER WHERE YOU GO, your experiences accompany you. Everyone has a past. It happened. It's in the recesses of our beautiful brains that God gives us. You can run, but you can't hide. Our pasts are always a part of us. And here's the thing;

You must deal with your past, or your past will control you.

Kathy and I both come from families that went far beyond dysfunctional. Perhaps our calling to South Africa was an unknown inner effort to get as far away from our childhoods as possible.

Sometimes unwittingly, we head off to a new place, traveling the farthest distance from point A—our pasts—to point B, our newly believed reality. For a time, our A becomes a remote, forgotten existence. Yet, it resurfaces when B slides back into A, melding two realities into one.

If your once upon a time was pleasant, good for you. Count your blessings. Remember those events when your present appears not so promising. But for many of us, whose pasts are littered with traumatic experiences, forgetting becomes a colossal fruitless effort at times. That's because we can never entirely forget our yesterdays. The past makes up our present.

Our pasts affect us both positively and negatively. Growing up with alcoholic parents, for example, fosters adverse childhood experiences (ACEs).[24] Children of alcoholics are much more likely to become addicted to alcohol or drugs. I've seen this firsthand.

Someone involved in a near-fatal car accident may fear getting into a vehicle. I had that conversation with a man two years ago. Involved in a horrible wreck, it took him many months before he summoned up the courage to drive again.

There are some experiences that you just can't shake off. Mental illness can quickly become our identity, but this is not accurate. A friend of mine—Jane—a counselor at Graceworks in Tyler, Texas, shared her thoughts:

> I often tell my clients that trauma or mental illness is not an identity. The reason is that sometimes, people get a 'secondary gain' from this identity and do not look for healing.
>
> For instance, the terms co-dependent or enabler seem to give people a handle on what drives their behavior, but they might use it as an excuse and, therefore, an identity.
>
> In school, they taught us not to say, 'So and so is Bi-polar' but rather, 'So and So has bi-polar.'
>
> Our identity is in Christ.[25]

Christ is my identifier. In weakness, like Paul in 2 Corinthians 12:8-10, my identity and purpose in Christ become clearer. With PTSD, I don't want it to become my identifier. It doesn't define me but motivates me to gain control over it. Then, I help others to do the same.

Learn to Deal With Your Past

Comatose realities buried deep within our minds can resurface. That episode—or thing you want to forget—occupies brain space.

That's because they are one.

You must deal with your past, or your past will control you.

Our past is our past.

You can't escape it.

You can try to ignore it.

Run from it.

But it's always there.

Disturbing events of childhood, inappropriate relationships, unwholesome habits, or mental deficits assail us.

Decide to deal with it. How? That may require reaching out for help.

It's a constant.

It's part of our being.

Part of who we are.

The past is part of the present.

Our pain can become gain, a part of our very being. We need an agent to apprehend and use to benefit ourselves and others. Pain can draw us nearer to God rather than distance us.

When we arrived in South Africa, Kathy and I thought we'd gotten far enough away to forget. However, we rediscovered our pasts as those wonderful Zulu people shared their worst experiences with us. Together, we hurt and tried to heal.

Embrace Your Past

Rather than playing Hide and Seek with the past, I've learned it's best to confront it. Look it straight in the eyes. Deal with it. Acknowledge what took place. Get help in learning to navigate your brain's ability to cope with trauma.

For most of my life, I failed to see God in any of the unpleasantries of childhood.

My response was, "God... where were you?"

Looking back, it's clear that God was present and cared about me. Not that God approved of the cruelty of it all. But I think God tracked with it, bringing purpose from its pain.

We must see God working in our pasts. To many, this is a hard point to sell. A universal question usually occurs;

Why?

Why God, did you let this happen to me?
Why weren't you there?
Why didn't you do this or that?
Why don't you care?

Christ frees us from hiding within our pasts.

Who's to Say God Doesn't Care?

Many times, my anger flared towards the Almighty. I concluded that God just didn't care about the immediacy of my troubles. However, now I think the opposite is true. Jesus identifies with our suffering. Rather than removing our anguish, Christ embraced it on the cross. He suffers with us.

This High Priest of ours **understands** our weaknesses, for *he faced all of the same testings we do*, yet he did not sin.

Hebrews 4:15 Emphasis Mine

This provides a meaningful purpose, even in pain. Christ's life and death show the ultimate effort to redeem us, to make us worthwhile again. To heal us. Everything we want to be rid of and start anew lies within Jesus. Reaching out, Christ frees me from hiding in my past. Oh, my past is still present, but it doesn't possess as much control over me now.

Jesus is our restorative, abundant life. He removes the effects of an injurious past, granting new life. For me, God has done and is doing everything possible to right this mess in humanity.

Causes of Suffering

God often receives blame for everything. But, perhaps, we as humans bring much of it upon ourselves.

Whoa! Hang on a minute! You just said what?

Hear me out.

In the Garden, God entrusted us to care for this planet. Humans are to be the stewards of this earth, but not only are we lousy at tending this garden, but we're also destroying it.

Pollution, global warming, and a host of other observations show a planet in great trouble. We stand on the verge of a nuclear holocaust determined by a few individuals. Countries continue to test nuclear weapons. Who's to say what effects this has upon our health? Maybe human practices have caused many diseases in the past few centuries?

Media overloads our minds with information far beyond our brain's design.

Destructive habits ruin our minds and bodies.

We eat too much, drink too much, put unhealthy substances into ourselves, and then when the obvious appears, ask, "Why Me?"

We bombard ourselves with the electromagnetic spectrum—waves of frequency—with every imaginable device from, microwaves to the internet, cell phones, and televisions. Yes, I own a cell phone and watch TV.

But how does pumping radiation from an artificially made device affect our health? What about the artificial chemicals in our foods? Our animal-based diets? No, I'm not a vegetarian. The altering of ecosystems?

How does all this affect us?

During the Black Plague in the 14th century, unsanitary practices aboard trading ships spawned the explosive growth of rats. Rats gave way to fleas. Once bitten by infected fleas, the plague spread rapidly through human populations.

Sometimes, ignorance is a culprit.

The cause of the Covid epidemic? Some postulate that it actually came from bats! We're not sure how it jumped to humans, but perhaps it's because of some human interference with the bat's ecosystem. Now, the CIA claims the virus came from a Chinese biological weapons lab.[26]

That car wreck that killed children often gets blamed on God rather than the drunk driver who crossed over the median, hitting a car head-on.

My FSHD Muscular Dystrophy is easy to blame on God, too. However, perhaps this genetic disorder's cause has nothing to do with God and everything to do with us? We just don't know, do we?

When someone exploits another? Where is God, then?

My mind ponders such questions.

The horrible things people do to others are hardly God's fault. We are violent beings bent towards war and self-destruction. It's within our nature to harm, control, enslave, and kill. If I'm going to be peeved, my anger is better directed towards the perpetrator, not God.

What this world needs is precisely what Jesus taught:

Love one another.
Love your neighbor like you; yourself want to be loved.
Forgive one another.
Forgive your enemies.

The Inexplicable

Many events occur in which there seems to be no answer to the question, "Why?"

When a tsunami kills thousands.

When a tornado destroys an elementary school in Oklahoma, killing children.

When a city bus driver goes into insulin shock, passing out at the wheel, driving his bus into an oncoming car, and killing the occupant inside.

When all those little kiddos with cancer enter St. Jude's Children's Hospital. Thank goodness for those wonderful people at St. Jude's!

From my years in South Africa, the countless sick children dying with no one to help them.

I'd like to think God cares. Has a plan for all of this. That's what faith is about, I guess. But in the areas I don't understand, it's difficult. This I admit. How can we come to any conclusions about God in such matters?

I find some common ground with Philip Yancey,

We may experience times of unusual closeness, when every prayer is answered in an obvious way and God seems intimate and caring.

And we may also experience 'fog times' when God stays silent, when nothing works according to formula, and all the Bible's promises seem glaringly false.

Fidelity involves learning to trust that, out beyond the perimeter of fog, God still reigns and has not abandoned us, no matter how it appears.[27]

Let God Into Your Past

I think we often lock God out of our hurts. Maybe it's because we don't feel that God cares. That he can't do anything about it, anyway. Or that we're not worthy of God's time. We become Christian agnostics, struggling with the wrongs affecting us.

I choose instead to allow God into my pain rather than ruminate about what I don't understand. Three verses from the Bible help me here. They come from Paul:

> Three different times I *begged* the Lord <u>to take it away</u>. Each time he said, '<u>My **grace** is all you need</u>. My power works best in weakness.'
>
> So now *I am **glad*** to [boast about my weaknesses,] so that the power of **Christ can work through me**.
>
> **That's why** *I take pleasure in my weaknesses*, and in the *insults, hardships, persecutions*, and *troubles* that I suffer for Christ. For *when I am weak*, then **I am strong**.
>
> 2 Corinthians 12:8-10 Emphasis Mine

Here, Paul was dealing with a painful issue. He went to God three times about it. When God refused to remove his pain, he came to three conclusions:

1. God's Promise

I am all you need. My grace—favor, and presence—is enough to get you through this. In me, you're an overcomer.

God promises never to leave or forsake us—he isn't walking away from us, leaving us stranded in our pasts. Hebrew 13:5, Isaiah 41:10

2. God's Presence

God is just as much a part of our past as we are. Theologically, we know God is everywhere. However, we struggle to sense God's presence in our pain.

Yet, we know God is with us even in the most troublesome moments, the most painful of memories. In this, we can take negative, harmful thoughts captive. We make them our prisoner, gaining control over our thinking process.

We demolish arguments and every pretension that sets itself up against the knowledge of God, and we take captive every thought to make it obedient to Christ.

2 Corinthians 10:5 NIV

3. God's Purpose

From my past, as troublesome as it was, I can now see God in it. While painful at the moment of impact, a troubled past can move us towards a meaningful purpose. 2 Corinthians 1:4 Pain becomes tolerable Upon finding purpose in our pain. And pain becomes productive.

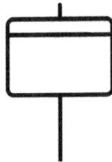

God and Your Past

Acknowledge the pain of your past. It's part of what makes you, you.

The most painful part of my past is _____?

I struggle to see God in _____?

In 2 Corinthians 12:8-10, I can most identify with _____?
Where do you see God in your past?

Like Paul, how can you take pleasure in your weakness?
Where does your past enable you?

When does Christ's power work through your weakness to help others?

Paul ends 2 Corinthians 12:10 by saying, "For when I am weak, then I am strong."

How might this apply to you? Finding strength in your weakness?

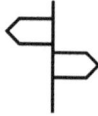

The Way Ahead

The past is part of our present. If not managed in the light of God's healing care, what becomes of us? Without God, our past adds enormous stress to living. Unmanaged stress derails health, relationships, and satisfaction with life. Unbridled stress ends up leading us rather than controlling it.

Part III

Mental Health Warning Signs

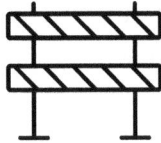

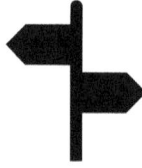

Guidepost #6

Unmanaged Stress Manages You

WHEN WAS THE LAST TIME you've spoken with a missionary who spent considerable time in the field that struggled with depression?

With a STRESSED-OUT pastor?

A church staff member?

That person sitting in church hiding their challenges in life?

The couple whose marriage is dying?

A single parent, struggling to raise a family?

Parents unable to get health care for their child?

Someone who has recently become homeless?

Seniors, after saving their entire lives, find themselves in need because of an explosive inflation rate that reduced their savings to almost nothing?

Or like me, as I began to write this book, diagnosed with a genetic disorder promising to strip me of my ability to comb my hair, button my shirt, or brush my teeth. As I struggle now to perform mundane tasks, stress sits next to me, uttering, "How's it going?"

What is Stress?

While it wears many faces, ***stress*** *simply is a sense of being overwhelmed by a situation in which you struggle to cope with its pressures.*

We all experience stress. It's a part of our daily existence. Short-lived periods of stress are normal, but *when chronic stress occurs for long periods, it becomes detrimental to health.*[28]

I think my mother's instability owed itself to awful levels of stress. This led to her drinking excessively. I remember many nights as the oldest child, still a little boy, sitting at the kitchen table with my mom crying, "What are we going to do?" Let's talk about missionary life again. That's the life I'm most familiar with. You may not be a missionary, but I think you can relate.

Missionary life fills itself with new relationships and unimaginable adventures. It also brings unprecedented levels of tension and strain. Stresses that few missionary candidates foresee or prepare for before leaving for their fields of service.

Upon hitting the tarmac at the airport, Sent Ones enter a land that doesn't expect them and rarely wants them. Dysfunctional missionary teams that don't get along often are the first to meet them. Many missionaries find themselves at an extreme disadvantage with little cognitive awareness of how to recognize or manage their new off-the-chart stress levels.

We entered South Africa in 1986. All my missionary companions told me it'd take months, perhaps a year, to install a phone. This was before cell phones and the internet. The amount of hoops and hurdles we jumped through just to get a PHONE. The forms we filled out, special letters from the home office in Missouri to verify that we needed phones, and going to Telkom's office in Ladysmith, South Africa, repeatedly ensured the phone arrived in record time; four weeks.

Enrolling our sons in school proved to be a herculean task, too. People in charge of transcripts didn't understand our sons' report cards and academic records. Just entering our son into kindergarten brought on a migraine.

Figuring out how to do anything was taxing. Where to rent a house, how to get utilities connected, setting up new bank accounts, and enrolling our sons in school for the first time presented unknown challenges. Just driving in South Africa initially was a hair-raising affair.

Learning the Zulu language marked more than a few hours of daily study. Even after two years, I could barely converse. And then, navigating the political unrest and rampant violence throughout the country had us constantly looking over our shoulders. To this day, now living in the United States, my situational awareness mimics the apprehensions of living in South Africa. I'm always looking over my shoulder. Danger hides everywhere.

Then, our biggest hurdle was trying to discover how to make friends in a country where everyone was a stranger and considered you even stranger. I realized that we were always outsiders regardless of how we wanted to meld ourselves into South African culture.

The demanding journey of leaving one's passport country, entering another culture, and beginning a new life pours crushing stress upon even the most dedicated. Only to be repeated upon returning to one's birth country. Bible training and internships that Western churches and missionary organizations offer little preparation for life after missionary service.

Upon returning 'home,' twenty years later, we found little in common with American Christians. Prayer meetings often addressed nonessentials. Church gatherings differed so much from our years in Africa that we felt like visitors. Eighteen years later, we still feel the same.

The busy American lifestyle overwhelmed us. Kathy and I felt like we couldn't catch our breath. And, as we tried to engage in conversations, we had little to offer that had anything in common with people. They often seemed to pull away from us.

One person, noting my struggle, offered advice over coffee. "Don, your conversations are always so serious, like life and death. People want to talk about things like their kids in school, their pets, and their favorite coffee shop, not about world hunger and poverty. The world is just not as serious a place to us as it is to you."

We learned quickly that few wanted to hear about our missionary lives any longer. What we'd spent our lives discussing in front of American audiences didn't matter now. In their eyes, we were no longer missionaries. But we couldn't separate twenty years of life and ministry in South Africa from our conversations. Those experiences will always be a part of us. Who we were and who we are. So, we had very little to talk about with the people we tried to connect with.

Just How Stressful is Life?

Years ago, while living in South Africa, I took the Holmes-Rahe Stress Scale. They developed the test in 1967 after examining the records of 5,000 medical patients to determine whether stressful events attributed to their illnesses. Patients took the test based on 43 life events and then relative score.[29] Each life event had a numerical score. Here are a few examples:

- Death of a spouse 100
- Death of a family member 63
- Personal injury or illness 53
- Business readjustment 39
- Change in responsibilities at work 29
- Change in residence 20
- Change in school 20
- Change in church activities 19
- Change in social activities 19

Stress is a killer lurking in our lives.

The results are then put in ranges:

- **150 points or fewer** | a relatively moderate amount of life change and a low susceptibility to stress-induced health breakdown.
- **150 to 300 points** | 50% chance of health breakdown in the next 2 years.
- **300 points or more** | 80% chance of health breakdown within the next 2 years, according to the Holmes-Rahe statistical prediction model.[30]

When I took my test, I scored over 700. That didn't include:

- The little Zulu girl who died in my arms from AIDS the following week.
- A friend gunned down in a robbery that month.
- My Neurologist in Pietermaritzburg, South Africa, poisoned to death two weeks later over a lover's quarrel.
- Having our pickup truck stolen the next month.

Most missionaries land high on the Holmes Rahe Stress Test, around 600. First-term missionaries can average as high as 900![31] There is justifiable criticism of the Holmes Rahe Stress Test. However, it's safe to assume that high—almost intolerable—stress levels exist among missionaries, but that doesn't mean they're the only ones who experience, at times, practically unbearable stress levels.

After coming off the field from South Africa, I accepted the lead pastor role at a medium-size church. There, with a Christian school, multiple staff to manage, and the three eight-member boards that ran the church, crushed me by adding new stressors.

Clergy members carry massive amounts of pressure. Balancing life, family, and overwhelming pastoral duties produces prolonged abnormal stress levels. Then, there are the few ecclesiastical terrorists in the congregation who believe their calling is to confront their pastor on every issue. These confrontations can trigger a fight or flight response.

The Search for Empathy

I remember back around 1995, trying to share with an adult Sunday school class in Wisconsin my extreme angst about witnessing people murdered in South Africa.

One woman piped up, "Oh, we always have that here. In Milwaukee, they murder people every day."

Milwaukee? A place an hour away from her location. A place she'd never visited nor dared step foot. Yet, she could identify with me? Such comparisons are often made in ignorance.

Again, attempting to share my difficulties with the sights, sounds, and smells of murder in South Africa, a pastor shot back, "The ministry is tough everywhere. Suck it up, buttercup." Sarcastically, I responded, "Right, how many members in your congregation had their fathers murdered and dismembered last year?"

I get grumpy sometimes.

His gems of wisdom offered in that exchange came while sitting in an eight-hundred-dollar office chair in an air-conditioned office, drinking a latte he made on his $2,000 barista coffee maker.

Yeah, his life looked tough.

But you know what? Observation over time showed a stress-filled life. He and his oldest son were estranged from each other. He hid his marriage problems. His daughter married, inviting her siblings but not Mom and Dad. They discovered the wedding on Facebook. Most staff members who quit working for him left bitter and remorseful. I felt sorry for him.

Can you relate?

Finding someone to share your harshest experiences is almost impossible. That's why:

Firefighters talk with firefighters about the fire scene.

ER nurses talk with ER nurses about what is happening in the emergency room.

Soldiers talk with soldiers about the battlefield.

Teachers talk with teachers about the classroom.

Missionaries talk with missionaries because they can understand missionary stress.

And that's why, as a pastor, I spoke with other pastors about pastoring. We talk with those we believe can relate to our situation without grasping that perhaps we need help beyond our friends.

Learn to Recognize Stress

Intermountain Healthcare gives some helpful advice on recognizing stress:

> Stress is a physical and emotional response to a situation. The situation may be positive, like a new baby or a job promotion. Or it can be negative, like a traffic jam or a fight with your teenager. Your body actually doesn't know the difference, it just knows that something is happening, and it should get ready to respond.[32]

We all experience it daily, but it's the long-protracted seasons that wear us down. How then are we to deal with stress? Many ways exist to tackle this demon. For me, a holistic, multi-pronged approach is best.

Avoid Excessiveness. Too much of any activity creates stress. Excessively involving yourself in a singular pursuit reduces time for other important considerations. While any pursuit may be good or neutral, a good thing becomes detrimental if it causes neglect in other important areas of life.

For instance, making a career your highest priority may require ignoring family or fitness.

Or an individual who's always at the fitness center. Workouts become a priority, above all other considerations. This reduces time spent on different activities to make room for the gym.

It's like how an addiction works. Whether an addiction to porn, online video gaming, use of computers, casino gambling, alcohol, tobacco, prescription drugs, work, opiates, fentanyl, food addictions, shopping addiction, thrill-seeking, fitness, TV, or whatever, addiction robs time from other functions of life.

When a substance, activity, or thing becomes a chronic harmful habit that alters our brain function—thinking, perspective, or attitude—an addiction is born.

Apart from the psychological ramifications of an addiction, it also affects our spiritual health. Christians I meet who are struggling with addictions rarely express a spiritually healthy disposition. Excessiveness spawns stress, then that stress dictates our lives in unhealthy directions.

Balance is the key. I've noticed that most stressed-out people often lack balance, ignoring critical life aspects.

A pastor friend attended monthly meetings with a dozen other pastors. Occasionally, I found time to pop into those small gatherings. In every meeting, he spoke of his relentless pursuit of his PhD in theology. He talked incessantly about the time he spent working on that degree.

Six months later, his wife served my friend with divorce papers. That was not only the end of his marriage. The church soon voted to dismiss him, leaving him unemployed. The very thing he gave himself to he lost.

Imbalances in our lives often require sacrifice of the best over good. Look at your life. How balanced are your passions and priorities versus nonessentials?

Your last physical? I CAN NOT emphasize this enough. Many times, Christians share what they believe is depression or some other mental ailment, only to find out their source of anxiety is more physical than mental.

The two connect, but sometimes, after treating a physical ailment, mental health improves. As one suffering from a long-term disabling genetic disorder, I know that physical health affects mental health. And as pastors, missionaries, and Christians, we often neglect our health.

Please pay attention to your physical health. Get that yearly checkup. Don't allow busyness to rob you of fitness. Make your physical health a priority. Stay on top of it.

How's your sleep? Sleep deprivation becomes debilitating when it's chronic and long-lived. Sleep-run-down people are simple to spot as they drag through life. Staying up all night, watching media, scrolling, and other nocturnal quests rob us of wellness.

Get plenty of sleep. If you're struggling, deal with it. See a doctor. Sleep is one of the best things we can do for ourselves.

How about a break from the News? News media worldwide often focus on the worst of the worst. One hundred years ago, most people only knew of events in their immediate proximity. They absorbed small bits and pieces of information.

Today, however, we overload our minds daily with multiple events worldwide, bombarding ourselves with continuous streams of traumatic information.

TIME recently ran an article; *Watching War Unfold on Social Media Affects Your Mental Health.* In it Ducharme says,

> Research suggests that news coverage of traumatic events can affect viewers' mental health—and with footage and photos from Ukraine flooding social media and misinformation spreading rampantly, that has implications for public health. [33]

Roxane Cohen Silver, a researcher on media coverage and trauma, says, "The amount of media someone consumes and how graphic that content influences mental health." [34]

"The best predictor for having lower anxiety and depressive symptoms was to avoid watching too much news," said Dr. Radua, a psychiatrist affiliated with King's College London and the Karolinska Institute in Sweden.[35]

Today, news outlets inundate us with thousands of bits and pieces of humanity's worst elements.

It's the same with social media. Do I really need to know what's going on in a dozen people's lives that I've never met and don't know?

Then there's rage news flooding social media. During the 2020 election, constant anger spilled out over people's Facebook posts. Whether Right or Left, people raged through social media. Give the news and social media periodic breaks.

Make time to unravel. Sometimes we wind ourselves so tightly the only result is pop!

Interestingly, the word 'wound' is from the old English word 'wund' and means 'ulcer' or 'injury.' Apparently, hundreds of years ago, being wund too tight was a problem too.[36]

When do you unwind? How do you unwind?

For me, listening to blues music helps calm my mind. Exercise always helps me unwind. Writing is my go-to place of respite. For Kathy, painting nature scenes with watercolors eases tension.

Find your calm place, and go there often.

Be Careful of over-isolation. During the Covid pandemic, we learned that long-term isolation is detrimental to mental health. Sometimes, those with mental health challenges withdraw into seclusion, shutting themselves off from friends and family. This leads to loneliness and disassociation. When you're alone, you're lonely because you're alone.

Missionaries and pastors often withdraw into seclusion. They retract themselves from everyday life, used up, worn out, and wound tight. I did this as a pastor. I attended to my duties, but afterward, I withdrew from everyone. That proved unhealthy for both Kathy and myself.

Simon and Garfunkel's hit song, *I Am a Rock*, ends with:

I am shielded in my armor
Hiding in my room, safe within my womb,
I touch no one and no one touches me
I am a rock. I am an island.
And a rock feels no pain
And an island never cries

Yes, a rock feels no pain, but people do. An island may never cry, but isolation, especially for those struggling with their mental health, is rarely sound. Social isolation often produces people with higher levels of depression and mental maladies. [37]

Recognize your need for help. Pastors and missionaries, we're the absolute worst sometimes in seeking help when in mental distress. Our constant stressful routines put us at a high risk. Yet, we don't understand or admit it.

Pastor, with our superhero, God-called-me thinking, we'd never stoop to admitting that an ultra-spiritual person like ourselves need help. What would people think? We're a little hypocritical here, don't you think?

Missionaries, we're no better. For us, with our bigger-than-life God-callings, we're not susceptible to mental health issues. Right? No, of course not. That's until we go off the rails into depression, anger, or other unhealthy expressions.

Loving Jesus while attending to spiritual challenges doesn't guarantee an unhindered life from mental challenges. Let's do better. Seek help when it's needed. Let's discipline and humble ourselves before God and people, making sure we don't become castaways from that which we've dedicated our lives. 1 Corinthians 9:27

Be discerning about who you ask for help, to those you invite into your inner circle, revealing your challenges. But get help. When we manage stress well, life becomes more navigable, lending itself to enjoyment and appreciation. Deal with your stress or surely it will deal with you.

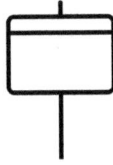

Take a Stress Test

Holmes Raye Life Stress Inventory

https://www.stress.org/wp-content/uploads/2024/02/Holmes-Rahe-Stress-inventory.pdf

Mindful Stress Test

Mental Health American–Stress Screener
https://www.bemindfulonline.com/test-your-stress

Mill Creek Christian Counseling
https://www.mhanational.org/get-involved/stress-screener

5 Ways to Reduce Stress

Heather Estep, MS, LMHCA
https://millcreekchristiancounseling.com/5-ways-to-reduce-stress/

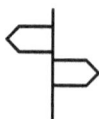

Where Does Stress Lead?

Unregulated stress controls us. It negatively affects our lives. I see this all the time. The person who's piled too many deadlines upon themselves. Sleep eludes them, pain pursues them, and people avoid them.

Then they ask themselves, "Why is this happening to me?"

Some stress is unavoidable. Some is self-inflicted. We need to admit that a lot of stress derives from our inability to recognize and regulate it. The result is often depression.

Unbridled stress becomes a catalyst for depression in many. For others, mental illness originates from epigenetic inheritance. This is a fixed inheritable observable characteristic resulting in changes to a chromosome without altering one's DNA, a propensity to be born with a trait towards mental health challenges.[38]

My mother struggled with depression, as did her mother. Hence, some of my depression may owe itself to epigenetic inheritance. What history of mental illness in your family might be affecting you?

Depression often sends out warning signs before its arrival. Recognition of these signs is key to dealing with it.

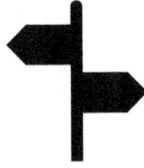

Guidepost #7

Depression Warns Before Its Arrival

Regular screening for depression and anxiety with early intervention are essential in ensuring good missionary health and productivity, though the missionaries themselves may find ways to cope or even refuse help. [39]

Find laughter. Find the smallest glimmers of joy. And chase them.

Gruver, Diana - Companions in the Darkness

WHEN 'FEELING DEPRESSED' TURNS INTO turns into long seasons of unhappiness, despair, sadness, misery, or hopelessness that won't go away, you're probably suffering from some level of depression.

Now, if you're of the mindset, like the lady who spoke with me last night after church, that 'spiritual' people—those who are really close to God—never get depressed or suffer from mental illness, then perhaps you'll skip this chapter. Or maybe, read the Bible a bit, for people struggling with depression fill its pages.

Depression: Out of the Will of God?

Once, while speaking to missionaries on *The Stresses of Missionary Life,* using Elijah's asking God to kill him as an example, a young missionary had something to say.[40] He blurted out, "I was taught that Elijah got depressed because he was out of the will of God."

I replied, "What was God's will for Elijah?"

Of course, nowhere in the Scriptures exists an emphatic statement that Elijah was 'out of God's will.' But like much of the Bible, we read what we want it to say in a passage.

Discussing this question resulted in an hour of facial expressions showing puzzlement. That's exactly what I hoped the question might accomplish. After extensively showing Elijah's expenditure of physical, emotional, and mental energy, then running from Queen Jezebel, and the stages of Elijah's suicidal ideation, most of the young missionaries still thought that Elijah's problem was that 'he was out of God's will.' No one could substantiate God's will for Elijah, but whatever the will of God was, Elijah was out of it.

Several years later, one of those young missionaries, now in his middle 30s, approached me. "I see what you meant about Elijah."

Getting the Right People to Help the Right People

A MK—Missionary Kid—now in his forties, shared with me a conversation that arose among the staff at his church where he worked.

A missionary from their church had just returned from West Africa. Struggling, he sought help from the counseling department of his church. During a church-wide staff meeting, pastors openly discussed the missionary's perplexing situation.

75

One pastor stated, "He claims he has PTSD after experiencing multiple shootings, and the continue threat of unrest. I think we're a little over our heads on this one. We need to find additional help. Someone who specializes in trauma, perhaps."

The MK on staff added, "Yes, that missionary experienced several assaults in the market square, he also suffered a hijacking as well, and well… you can only imagine."

He continued, "It sounds like some of the stuff my dad experienced in Africa, and what we saw growing up as kids on the mission field. It's very difficult to deal with, personally, as I still struggle with some of it now."

With that, a biblical counselor on staff found a therapist skilled in helping trauma-ridden people. In fact, the therapist worked with many military veterans from the Iraq and Afghanistan wars who returned home with complex trauma issues.

A chief duty of a counselor is to listen to the counselee. Here, a very compassionate staff listened to this missionary. Finding him the help he needed, they aided this missionary in improving his mental health. And guess what? That missionary is back out in the field today.

It's the same with another missionary living with Attention-deficit/hyperactivity disorder (ADHD). Listening to him talk about his lifelong affliction, he mentioned a pastor who'd help him with his guilt at having to take medication.

"Without my medication," he began, "I become pretty dysfunctional after a few days. Mood swings, anger, and depression become immense problems for me. Pastor _____ helped me understand that my mental illness is not a faith deficit, and taking my medication is not a sin, but a wise necessity."

We must stop seeing mental illness as a faith deficit, denying its existence. Yes, indeed, spiritual components exist. However, understanding the brain's anatomy and its function convinced me that some types of depression exist outside of faith or lack thereof. Until we acknowledge faith as only part of the picture of mental health, mentally challenged people will continue to distance themselves from the Church.

> *We must stop seeing mental illness as a faith deficit.*

Sadly, the secular world of psychology often holds to a higher standard of mental health care and confidentiality than some biblical counselors.

It's crucial to vet church counselors to determine their expertise and ability to counsel, the counseling they're qualified to offer, and a policy of referring counselees to other mental health professionals when a patient requires help beyond our ability to give it. It's essential we recognize when we're over our heads lacking the training to deal with certain mental illnesses.

Depressed People in the Bible

While never using our modern word 'depression,' the Bible contains many stories of crippling depression. We find an excellent example in Nehemiah 2:2 when King Artaxerxes asked Nehemiah, serving as the King's Cup Bearer, "Why do you look sad? If you are not sick, *you must be sad at heart.*"

Nehemiah's depression developed over the state of his nation, people, and future. His disposition so overpowered him he couldn't hide it in a sad, disconsolate mood. Standing before the King demanded accolades and service. Failure to do so often resulted in death in the ancient world. Nehemiah's mood threatened his very life.

He was *sad at heart*... a heart sickness which sullied his mood, attitude, and behavior.

Another example of depression is that of Hannah. Depressed with her inability to bear children, her husband asks, "Why do you weep, and why do you not eat, and why is *your heart sad?*" 'Heart' is the Hebrew word for 'mind,' where thoughts and feelings—emotions—come from. So, "sad of heart" may point to mental illness.[41] 1 Samuel 1:8 NASB

What about Job? Did he suffer from depression? Several phrases in Job 33:19-22 indicate a deep despair. Elihu describes:

Man is also rebuked with pain on his bed and with continual strife in his bones, so that his life loathes bread, and his appetite the choicest food. His flesh is so wasted away that it cannot be seen, and his bones that were not seen stick out. His soul draws near the pit, and his life to those who bring death.

Job 33:19-22 ESV

The ASV translates verse nineteen:

He is chastened also with pain upon his bed, And with *continual strife in his bones.*"'Strife in the bones' portrays an image of extreme agitation and continual conflict that causes sleep disturbances. The extreme loss of interest in normal activities when someone is bedridden." [42]

The Book of Psalms is loaded with song singers☐worship leaders—describing their mental plight or that of others. The genre saturates worship with lamenting. Lamenting is considered in some contexts as depression.[43]

Here are just a few:

You **don't** let me **sleep**.
I am too **distressed** even to pray!
I think of the good old days,
long since ended,

when my nights were filled with joyful songs.
   I search my soul and ponder the difference now.
Has the Lord **rejected me** forever?
   Will he **never again** be kind to me?
Is his unfailing love **gone forever**?
   Have his promises permanently **failed**?
Has God **forgotten** to be gracious?
   Has he **slammed the door** on his compassion?

   ☐Asaph in Psalm 77:4-9 Emphasis Mine

The Korites, descendants of the Levites—a priestly class—wrote this Psalm during their exile in either Assyria or Babylon after they lost their country, homes, incomes, and families.

Day and night I have **only tears** for food,
   while my enemies continually **taunt me**, saying,
'Where is this **God** of yours?'
 My **heart is breaking**
   as I remember **how it used to be**:
Why am I **discouraged**?
   Why is my heart so **sad**?

☐Descendants of Korah in Psalm 42:3-4 & 43:5 Emphasis Mine

You have fed us with *sorrow* and made us drink tears by the bucketful.
   Psalms 80:5 Emphasis Mine

King Solomon talked about depression, "*Anxiety* in the heart of man causes *depression…*" Proverbs 12:25 NKJV Emphasis Mine

Then there is **David**—the Giant Slayer—who shared transparently his bouts with depression:

79

Save me, O God,
  for the **floodwaters are up to my neck**.
Deeper and deeper I **sink into the mire**;
  I **can't find** a foothold.
I am in **deep water**,
  and the **floods overwhelm** me.
I am **exhausted** from crying for help;
  my throat is parched.
My eyes are **swollen with weeping**,
  waiting for my **God to help** me.
Those who **hate me** without cause
  outnumber the hairs on my head.
Many enemies try to **destroy me** with lies,
  demanding that I give back what I didn't steal.

Psalm 69:1-4

Elijah, after extending all his energy spiritually, emotionally, and physically, cried out,

"… I've **had enough**, Lord," he said. "**Take my life**, for I am no better than my ancestors who have **already died**." I Kings 19:4

We try to spiritualize Elijah's depression as a temporary moment of discouragement. A close read of 1 Kings 18 & 19 finds a frayed prophet who laid bankrupt of strength and a willingness to live after expelling all his energy. He wanted to end it all; "God, take my life."." What was God's response? *Eat, drink, and get some rest. Then let's talk.*

King Saul exhibited significant signs of depression, too. I think two words summed up Saul's problem: *work* and *focus*. The work of leading Israel as its

80

first King carried huge stressors. After Saul failed his performance review with the Prophet Samuel, he focused on that which he could no longer have; the succession of his son serving on the throne.

Saul exhibited extreme paranoia. His life-threatening variations of behavior, long-seasoned melancholy moods, extreme manic episodes, irrational moods, and jealousy towards David all pointed to a King who suffered from mental illness. Some suggest he suffered from epilepsy, too.[44]

Amnon, the son of David, fell into depression because of his despairing lust for Tamar. "Amnon became so obsessed with Tamar that he became ill… Amnon thought he could never have her." 2 Samuel 13:2 Here, willful sin brought on Amnon's depression.

King Hezekiah lay ill. God instructed him to inform the family of his impending death. He showed signs of mental health decline in his uncontrolled crying. Isaiah 38:3

Ahab's depression included loss of appetite, withdrawal, a turning of his face towards the wall—a loss of interest in life. 1 Kings 21:4-5 His depression resulted from deep-seated sin as well.

Jeremiah's depression was real:

> My own **people laugh** at me.
>   All day long they sing their **mocking** songs.
> He has **filled me with bitterness**
>   and given me a **bitter cup** of sorrow **to drink**.
> He has made me **chew on gravel**.
>   He has **rolled me in the dust**.
> Peace has been **stripped away**,
>   and I have **forgotten** what prosperity is.

I cry out, "My **splendor is gone!**
Everything I had hoped for from the Lord **is lost**
The thought of my **suffering and homelessness**
    is **bitter beyond words.**
I will **never forget** this awful time,
    as I **grieve over my loss.**
            ☐Lamentations 3:14-20 Emphasis Mine

Again, we can spiritualize Jeremiah's words, making them not mean what they say. Yet, his bouts with depression are clear. Pushed to his mental edge in the suffering and brutality he witnessed, his acuity declined.

Jeremiah saw the murder of family and friends, the destruction of his home, and the ruin of the entire nation. Added to this was the death of the last righteous king of Judah.

Jeremiah's warnings in 601 BC saw the downfall and destruction of everything he owned and valued. Yet, he still served God during this miserable condition. Living in Jerusalem and Egypt for the rest of his life, he enjoyed no home or country to call his own.

I can relate to Jeremiah a bit. The ruthless violence witnessed during my twenty-plus years in South Africa still carries images unvanquished in my mind.

We could talk about **Johan, Moses, Naomi, Joseph,** Depression is real. It's often affected God's people. *I did not say it affects all of God's people,* but it is, unfortunately, a part of our fallen condition. Sometimes, as mentioned, sin is a contributing factor to depression, but it is not always or only THE factor for an individual's depression symptoms.

Influential Christian Leaders

We like to highlight the successes of historic Christian leaders. Yet, many of the movers and shakers of Christianity's past suffered bouts of severe manic depression.

Martin Luther, the Father of the Reformation writhed in depression much of his adult life. Luther struggled with an inner turmoil and depressive angst he called in German *anfechtung*.[45] This challenging of the will, or 'temptation,' assailed him from the earliest days of his monastic life. Luther, aware of his sinful unworthiness, believed his soul was damned. He wrote in his journal:

"I lost touch with Christ the Savior and Comforter, and made him the jailer and hangman of my poor soul." [46]

Luther's friend and longtime mentor Johann von Staupitz advised, *"Look to the wounds of Christ,"* after giving him a Bible. [47]

I like Diana Gruver's words here:

So in the midst of depression, when we fall under the harassment of guilt and shame, we can follow Staupitz's advice as well. Look to the wounds of Christ. For this is where we see the extent of God's love, the upside-down way he brings beauty and wholeness, the full measure of his grace. It is where we are reminded of truth outside of our feelings—that nothing can separate us from God's love, not even the deepest depression.

Luther's life tells us this: the wounds of Christ will guide us through the darkness. [48]

Letters to his friends tell a story of a bleak and depressed inner person. Luther wrote his friend Philip Melanchthon,

'… despised worm that I am, vexed with a spirit of sadness.' [49]

83

Diana Gruver notes Luther's healthy response:

And yet he called this experience 'school.' As horrifying as his psychological state was, as much as he would have preferred death to the doubts and fears attacking his mind, Luther found that the experience taught him something. This trial, as with all others, was a schoolyard, a training ground. He would say elsewhere that trials make us more sure of doctrine, increase our faith, and teach us Scripture's true meaning.[50]

It's about this time Luther wrote his famous hymn *A Mighty Fortress is Our God.*

Luther encouraged:

Whenever the devil pesters you with these thoughts, at once seek out the company of men, drink more, joke and jest, or engage in some other form of merriment.[51]

That's excellent advice. Find friends who uplift your spirits. Put yourself in places that make you happy and healthy.

Luther continued:

The worst and saddest things come to mind. We reflect upon all sorts of evils. And if we have encountered adversity in our lives, we dwell upon it as much as possible, magnify it, think that no one is as unhappy as we are, and imagine the worst possible consequences.[52]

Charles Haddon Spurgeon—considered 'The Prince of Preachers' in many Evangelical circles—suffered from depression most of his life. He pastored a 19th-century mega-church in London. Writing prolifically and delivering his most excellent sermons, he wrestled with his deep depression.

He wrote:

'Sometimes you cannot raise your poor depressed spirits,' he said. Some say to you, 'Oh! you should not feel like this.' They tell you, 'Oh! you should not speak such words, nor think such thoughts.' Ah! the heart knows its own bitterness, and a stranger meddles not therewith—ay, and I will improve upon it, nor a friend either. It is not easy to tell how another ought to feel and how another ought to act.[53]

Once, while preaching to over 10,000 people, someone yelled, 'Fire!' The result of panicking people took 7 lives, leaving 28 other people in critical condition. For a few days afterward, Spurgeon remained in a dazed state. Eventually, he recovered, but the depths of depression never left him.[54] Even then, Spurgeon sought to understand those suffering from mental illness:

Let us be very tender with brethren and sisters who get into that condition. I have heard some say, rather unkindly, 'Sister So-and-so is so nervous, we can hardly speak in her presence.'

Yes, but talking like that will not help her; there are many persons who have had this trying kind of nervousness greatly aggravated by the unkindness or thoughtlessness of friends. [55]

In one of his sermons, he assured those suffering from depression that they were not the first to face such battles. He mentioned Isaac Newton, Robert Boyle, William Cowper, and a host of other contemporaries of that day. He continued:

There are times when our spirits betray us, and we sink into darkness. We slip into the 'bottomless pits' where our souls 'can bleed in ten thousand ways, and die over and over again each hour.' There is no reasoning, and a remedy is hard to find.[56]

Yet, Spurgeon gave witness to our ultimate hope:

Do not, therefore, think that you are quite alone in your sorrow. Bow your head, and bear it, if it cannot be removed; for but a little while and every cloud shall be swept away, and you, in the cloudless sunlight, shall behold your God.[57]

Lottie Moon, famed 19th century Southern Baptist single missionary in China, once wrote, "I pray that no missionary will ever be as lonely as I have been." [58]

Highly educated, she did something that few missionaries ever accomplished. Lottie mastered the Chinese language.

Through the Woman's Mission Union, she laid the foundation for raising millions of dollars annually for Southern Baptist Missions.

In all her accomplishments, she struggled with immense depression. After four years, with no help on the horizon, she wrote, "I am bored to death living alone. I don't find my own society either agreeable or edifying... I really think a few more winters like the one just past *would put an end to me. This is no joke, but dead earnest.*"[59]

Seeing the breakdown of other missionaries' mental, physical, and spiritual well-being, she advocated for long rest periods. Perhaps the practice of missionary furloughs found its beginning with Lottie. She practiced her own advice, often taking long breaks in other parts of China for rest, recuperation, and reentering her ministry.

Mother Teresa struggled with loneliness and depression. She wrote:

Oh, Absent One, how long will You stay away? I long for You, but You do not want me. Emptiness. Pain. Loneliness. I cannot express this pain. This is what hell is like—without God—no love, no faith. The pain is so great I feel as if everything will break. Who am I that You would forsake me? [60]

During my readings about Mother Teresa and her Sisters of Charity, I supposed her mental sufferings were equal to her amazing successes. She received international praise—something she never sought—receiving the Nobel Peace Prize. Yet underneath her beautiful, wrinkled skin lived an emotionally desolate person. She wrote again:

Lord, my God, who am I that You should forsake me? The child of Your love—and now become as the most hated one—the one You have thrown away as unwanted—unloved. I call, I cling, I want—and there is no One to answer—no One on Whom I can cling—no, No One.—Alone.

So many unanswered questions live within me—I am afraid to uncover them—because of the blasphemy. If there be God, please forgive me. Trust that all will end in Heaven with Jesus.

Love—the word—it brings nothing. I am told God loves me, and yet the reality of darkness & coldness & emptiness is so great that nothing touches my soul.[61]

President Abraham Lincoln suffered many bouts of melancholy. So, too, Thomas Jefferson, James Madison, Franklin Pierce, John Quincy Adams, and Calvin Coolidge experienced bouts of depression.[62] Martin Luther King battled depression. J. K. Rowling, the author of the Harry Potter series, suffered two bouts of depression.

Missionaries and Pastors Get Depressed, Too

A study by the Rosemead School of Psychology published in the *Journal of Psychiatry & Theology in 2015* looked at Missionary Health Care Workers during their tenures on the fields.

Survey respondents worked in 67 countries representing most regions of the world, including male and female participants. These individuals reported an average of 11 years of service, intending to continue to serve until retirement.

All the participants in this study were career missionaries employed by organizations whose primary purpose was selecting and training personnel for long term cross-cultural service. Self-reported depression severity scores of 3 or greater out of 5 comprised 55.5% of female and 45.0% of male participants' responses. Participants (10.47% of females and 15.34% of males) reported experiencing no depression.[63] That means, there are a lot of missionaries struggling with depression and anxiety.

Clergy rates of depression are twice that of the national average in the United States.[64] More than 1 out of 5 pastors have struggled with mental illness.[65] In an exception to the disability laws in the United States, Christian pastors and missionaries can lose their jobs because of their mental health status.[66] And they often do.

When Depression is Not Only a Spiritual Issue

Is all depression a result of sin? Well, yes, in the sense that we live in a sin-marred world handed down to us through Adam's disobedience. Romans 5:12 I've often thought about my first words to Adam upon seeing him in Eternity. Perhaps one word, "WHY!?"

Definitely, wrongdoing or willful sin can cause enough mental anguish to induce depression. We've noted many examples in Scripture pointing towards this. But there's another source of sin besides personal, willful sin.

Some depression arises from sin perpetrated upon us. As a victim attempts to live with the scars placed upon them by another, depression often follows. I know this firsthand with my PTSD.

Certain attitudes and moods I struggled with in the beginning stages of PTSD brought images of my mother grappling with the same emotional struggles. Those emotional struggles played out on us through harsh verbal language and physical abuse. As much as I didn't like it, I saw my mom in me.

Depression may arise from family history, illness, medical issues, substance abuse, medications, or personality. It's often a condition that doesn't have one specific cause.[67]

It would be a great oversight to assume every depressed person suffers from spiritual maleficence. Christ modeled a much more humanizing approach when reaching out to hurting people.

What Exactly then is Depression?

Mayo Clinic defines depression as:

A mood disorder that causes a persistent feeling of sadness and loss of interest. Also called major depressive disorder or clinical depression, it affects how you feel, think and behave and can lead to a variety of emotional and physical problems. You may have trouble doing normal day-to-day activities, and sometimes you may feel as if life isn't worth living.[68]

Depression affects more than just the mood; it affects the body too. A holistic approach to dealing with depression requires treating the entire person, not just one part of it.

When Depression Approaches

There are many signs of depression. Sometimes, they show up as just being a little down and out. Other times, it points towards major mental health issues. When depression approaches:

Change your routines.
Take a break.
Take the weekend off.
Take a vacation.
Go somewhere with the family.

Depression affects the entire person; mind, body, and soul.

89

Find a listening, empathetic ear.

Plan for a personal spiritual retreat to immerse yourself in prayer, God's Word, and a quieting of your mind.

Exercise.

Listen to soothing bilateral music.

Listen to Chopin, Vivaldi, and other classical composers. The Four Seasons Violin Concerto is one of my favorites.

Get a physical.

How about a massage? Try it! It might surprise you how much it helps.

Find something that makes you smile.

Laugh!

Control your media exposure.

Take a break from the news.

Learn to enjoy God. "How, you ask?" Well, that's the adventurous part. Search, discover, and enjoy!

Signs depression has become a mental health issue:

- ✓ You're tired all the time.
- ✓ Interrupted sleep patterns from night terrors or worry.
- ✓ Not enough or too much sleep.
- ✓ Indifference to life.
- ✓ Withdrawing and isolating yourself from those closest to you: family, spouse, team members, supporters, etc.
- ✓ Emotional Outbursts.
- ✓ A hyper-critical spirit about anything, everything, anybody, or everybody.
- ✓ Frequent illnesses.
- ✓ Sudden changes in habits and activities.
- ✓ Irrational purchases, selling, or disposing of items.

✓ Abnormal changes to diet, travel, or sexual desires.
✓ Inability to make decisions.
✓ Lack of concentration.
✓ A feeling of uselessness, hopelessness, or apathy.
✓ Dark moods.
✓ Suicidal Ideation.
✓ Feeling unhappy, alone, and empty.
✓ A loss of interest in all activities. "I just want to do nothing."

Now, as I understand, no one sign here means you suffer from depression. However—please get this—if five or more signs are evident, especially the last three, pay attention and get some help.

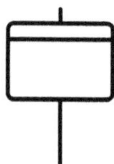

Positive Ways of Handling Your Depression

Let others into your life. We often attempt to go it alone. It's a sure path to defeat. King Solomon advised:

A person standing alone can be attacked and defeated, but two can stand back-to-back and conquer. Three are even better, for a triple-braided cord is not easily broken.

Ecclesiastes 4:12

Find people who will speak truth into your life with an empathetic ear. We often slog it out with a stubborn plow forward, no-matter-what-the-cost attitude. Or, we withdraw into a cocoon of gloom.

Some of the best people I didn't appreciate then were straight talkers with me. Compassionate truth speakers attempted to warn me of what was unfolding before them, but unbeknown to me.

Dave—a South African—brought to my attention a troublesome downturn in my person. Years later, that led to my diagnosis of PTSD. I resisted Dave's advancing observations. You know what? Dave was right, and though he died a year later at a Retreat Center outside of Escourt, South Africa, perhaps in heaven, I'll acknowledge that to him.

Listen to your spouse, family, friends, and coworkers. You may not want to hear it, but they see you from the outside in. As individuals, we tend to view ourselves from the inside out.

Find refreshing places. Jesus often dealt with vast crowds of pressing people during a hectic, busy ministry. Yet, we see our wonderful Savior slipping away to secluded places during a hectic, demanding ministry.

Seek a solitude of relaxation, reflection, and retrospection. Find a place to recharge. Visiting it often. Snatch opportunities to go somewhere quiet. Sit in prayer. Meditate. Reflect. Relax.

Here's Jesus' example, "… Jesus often withdrew to lonely places and prayed." Luke 5:16 NIV Want to be like Jesus? Rest.

Get some exercise. Here, my hypocrisy rears its head a bit. Exercise is a struggle for me, especially with my Facioscapulohumeral Muscular Dystrophy (FSHD).

Declining ability to move my arms and shoulders presents challenges. I hate exercising because it's painful. Everything hurts. So, I'll walk up and down the stairs. Walk the parking lot of the church. I follow a daily exercise routine by my physical and occupational therapists.

Exercise can be just a simple practice of moving. Here are a few ideas:

- Go for a walk.
- Mow the lawn.
- Play the guitar. Playing an instrument burns a ton of calories. Even with my FSHD Muscular Dystrophy, using a sling to hold up my right arm, I can still play the guitar or bass for an hour at a time.
- Take up gardening.
- Start a gym membership. Then go to the gym often.
- Maybe, hire a trainer.
- Go to the market.
- Dance.
- Throw a frisbee.
- Take the stairs rather than the elevator. Walk up the escalator rather than just standing.
- Park in a spot far from the door of the store you're entering. This forces you to walk.
- Take up hiking.
- Master the jump rope.
- Swim.
- Practice balancing.
- Deep clean your home, office, or church. Probably not a favorite choice here.
- Boxercize. Google it.
- Start riding a bike.
- Take up slacklining.
- Try the 10-Minute Workout.
- Get an exercise bike.
- Buy a treadmill.
- What about rock climbing?
- Wrestle with your kids. They need your time; you need the exercise.
- Martial Arts?

- Golf. Yes, it's expensive, so try mini-golf if you can't do that.
- Shopping. Yes, but go to the mall rather than online shopping.
- Play video games that make you active.
- How about building something? Put a fence up. Build a dollhouse. Repair that leaky faucet.
- Jumping jacks.
- Shoot baskets with the kids.
- Try the Couch Potato Workout.
- Suck your stomach in and tighten your abs while sitting on the couch or in the car at a red light. Hold the position for five seconds. Repeat five to ten times per day.
- Stand on one leg.
- Work your inner thighs while sitting on the couch.
- Leg raises.
- Put a folded pillow between your legs. Bring your thighs together, pressing upon the pillow for a few seconds, and then release.
- Use your imagination.
- Discipline yourself towards movement rather than physical stagnation.
- *The important thing is to get up and move. Get going.*

See a Therapist. There are good Christian therapists out there who specialize in specific disciplines of mental health. For me, seeing a trauma therapist was a lifesaver.

Tom, a licensed therapist in Minnesota, focused on helping me alter my emotions and thoughts resulting from traumatic experiences. This helped me control my responses to those experiences. He recommended further treatment.

I began seeing a new therapist after moving to Texas. Jane started treating me using EMDR—Eye Movement, Desensitized, and Reprocessing. It was only after EMDR that my sleep improved. For the first time in fifteen years, I began sleeping through the night at least four times per week. Up till then, I rarely slept more than four hours per night.

Finding a therapist that's a good fit is often a daunting task. Your mental health, however, is worth it. Several good networks list certified Christian therapists. Check out sites like: https/www.aacc.net/International Board of Christian Care, https:/www.ibccglobal.com/find-a-provider/

Take medication? Your doctor might recommend taking psychotropic medication. I'm not of the camp that believes it's a sin to take such medications. That's no truer than it's a sin to take Tylenol for a migraine.

The common underhand accusation is, "It's a lack of faith or sin to take medication for mental health." Tell me, where is that statement clearly supported in Scripture?

Another accusation comes, "Well! There's so many unpleasant side effects."

Yes, that's possible. Yet, the side effects from my heart medication don't wave me off all other medications. It means changing from one pill to another until we find a medication that improves my heart function with minimal side effects. Any medication for anything may cause side effects.

Sure, there's an argument to be made, especially in the United States, that we're an overmedicated society. I'm only saying to take what you need when you need it, and no more. Always follow your doctor's advice.

Caution Here. Be informed about the mental health drugs you're taking. They can affect you adversely, causing side effects and suicidal or violent thoughts. Contact your health provider immediately about such might occur.

Seek Help. This is the most important step. One of the wisest wrote, "… in the multitude of counsellors there is safety." Proverbs 11:14 KJV Find someone to trust and confide in.

Find people who will speak truth into your life with an empathetic ear.

95

Yes, it's always a risk to confiding in someone else. People rarely keep confidence. But good mental health is worth the risk.

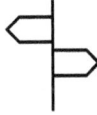

Other Culprits of Poor Mental Health

While depression can play huge detrimental roles in our mental health, another culprit may take a more significant toll on us: anger.

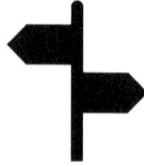

Guidepost #8

Uncontrolled Anger Controls You

I suppose there is nothing more damaging our Christian lives than uncontrolled anger, for it ends many beginnings.

A SOUTH AFRICAN friend, Keith, pointed out my anger to me. "You always seem to get angry at any mention of your father." We'd shared a bit of our history over a cup of tea, trying to get acquainted. Then Keith talked about his dad.

He and his father farmed together in Witbank, South Africa, just southwest of Kruger National Park. He shared many pleasant memories of living next to his family and farming together until farm life became too dangerous. The killing of white farmers forced them to give up their farm and buy a BP Gas Station in Ladysmith. They moved in next to us on Hyde Road. "It was a wonderful time of life," Keith concluded.

With that, I blurted out unintentionally, "Good for you." The comment was strong and naively angry.

"Don, did I say something wrong?" Keith queried.

"No, sorry, I just didn't enjoy that kind of father," I replied.

As Keith and I became exceptional friends, he gently marked my below-the-skin seething antagonism at the mentioned fatherhood. He helped me see my unchecked anger.

Violence marked the home we grew up in. My father perpetrated much of that for the first ten years of my life until he left. After that, Mom loved us, but alcohol and the pressures of single parenting often got the best of her, turning our home into a nightmare at times.

During the 1960s, few homes were as fatherless as they are today. Back then, Dad's departure from a familial relationship marked us. Often, biting comments came from classmates at school about our fatherless plight. The tongue is such a weapon of emotional destruction, isn't it?

Whenever other fathers interacted with their children, storms of emotions welled up. As a young teenager, I remember sitting on the stairway many times during the early hours of the weekends. Watching the car lights down the dark road, hoping my father would stop, step out of the car, and hug me.

Innocently, this produced an immense amount of resentment. That anger accompanied me to South Africa.

Unchecked Anger is Unhealthy

At a church in Ladysmith, South Africa, where I spoke many times, an inebriated man entered the property during a Sunday afternoon church gathering. He, being from a different ethnic group, incurred the wrath of the leaders of that 'Evangelical Bible Church.'

When the sozzled man refused to leave, four 'Christian' men who learned martial arts as young children went into a frenzy. The black man resisted. The four Indian men killed him.

Every killing I've ever witnessed in South Africa was fueled by anger; alcohol and drugs usually accompanied the bloodletting as well. With most violent events wreaking havoc, anger is often the catalyst.

Christians are not exempt. Angry people sit amid our liturgies, worship, music, Scripture reading, and sermons. It surprises me the many hostile church attendees, missionaries, and pastors I've met. It shouldn't be. I've carried such hostilities myself. Angry people fill our churches. Anger directs our conversations. It directs attitudes and interactions with others. Anger permeates the soul.

Living in the United States and spending twenty-plus years in South Africa attests that anger is a mainstay of our human existence. People are angry about anything, everything, and nothing.

Occasionally, someone shares, "I'm angry all the time. I wake up and go to bed angry." Solomon, the wisest sage, talked about this type of anger:

> People ruin their lives *by their own foolishness* and then **are angry at the Lord**. Proverbs 19:3 Emphasis Mine

We are solely responsible for our own uncontrolled anger.

God often receives blame for our anger. Somehow, our misfortunes and destructive behavior become God's fault. It's common to be angry with God.

God, why me?
Why did that happen?
Why am I sick?
Why did they do that to me?
Why did my spouse leave me?
Why did you let me lose my job?
Why don't people like me?
Why, after Covid, am I still sick, depressed, and tired?
Why, why, why…

King David, in his darkest hours, asked,

> My God, my God, why have you abandoned me?
> Why are you so far away when I groan for help?

Psalm 22:1

The whys often hold God or others culpable for perceived injustices. It's here we validate our anger. Yet, we carry the sole responsibility for our own unrestrained anger.

A question might be, "What am I doing about my anger?" And "Nothing" shouldn't become the option. Anger brings echoing damage.

> Hot-tempered people must **pay the penalty**. If you rescue them once, you have to do it again.

Proverbs 19:19

But anger is a natural, God-given emotion. It can help us deal with the injustices and maladies of life, bringing about positive results. However, anger needs to be channeled and controlled.

Anger

Anger is difficult to define. The *American Heritage Dictionary* calls it "a strong feeling of displeasure or hostility."

I like Chip Ingram's definition, "We define anger as a charged, morally neutral, emotional response of protective preservation." [69]

Anger is neither good nor bad. Though anger is full of energy and can make our hearts pound as beads of sweat roll off our heads, it's really morally neutral unless… it goes unchecked.[70]

Anger is a God-given emotion, a gift. Its goal is to preserve and protect us or others when emotionally or physically threatened. While it can provide safety, anger in the wrong context leaves a backlash of injury, damage, and broken relationships.

Anger's Physiology

The brain's prefrontal cortex is behind the forehead. Divided into three parts, it forms the rational center of our brain. Fully developed around thirty years of age, this part of the brain involves personality characteristics, decision-making, and movement.[71] This part also **controls** anger.

People struggling with depression, schizophrenia, or bipolar disorder, to name a few, suffer dysfunction and dysregulation in at least one of three region areas of the prefrontal cortex: dorsolateral, ventrolateral, or the ventromedial prefrontal cortex, also known as the orbitofrontal PFC.[72]

When a person exhibits reckless behavior, this may result from injury to the orbital prefrontal cortex. When apathetic and unmotivated, doctors sometimes look at the medial prefrontal cortex for injuries. If a person cannot switch from one task to another, perhaps it's because the lateral prefrontal cortex has suffered damage.[73,74]

The emotional part of the brain is in the limbic system. This system is located under the temporal lobe in the cerebrum. Within the limbic system exist two small walnut-shaped organs called the amygdala. The amygdala marks the emotional center of our brains. Kayt Sukel notes:

This pair of almond-shaped organs deep within the brain help regulate emotion and encode memories—especially in more emotional remembrances.

We often think of the amygdala as being a sort of survival-oriented brain area. Things that have strong emotions associated with them, good and bad, are likely to be the things that allow a species to not only stay alive, but also thrive in its environment. Recent research, though, suggests that

101

the amygdala's role in memory consolidation may go beyond just the emotional aspects of our experiences.[75]

The amygdala **processes** and **expresses emotions**. This is especially true with anger and fear. The amygdala is always on the lookout for times of danger. It also carries the task of **helping us survive with fight, flight, freeze or flop responses to danger**.[76]

This part of the brain fully develops fully by the time we reach eight to ten years of age. That's why childhood trauma plays such huge detrimental roles in our lives as adults. What happens to us as children stays buried in our emotional brains, often resurfacing in our adult years.

Our rational brain—the prefrontal cortex—helps control our emotions. The problem is that often, anger or fear surrenders to the amygdala, allowing emotions to incapacitate us. We isolate in fear, freeze with shock, flop and switch off, or detonate through anger. As this happens, the prefrontal cortex sits uninvolved on the sidelines watching the home team go down in another lopsided loss.[77]

Both the prefrontal cortex and amygdala carry the same goal; helping you survive. The prefrontal cortex wants to plan complex cognitive behaviors, regulating our thoughts, actions, and emotions, but *often the amygdala's emotions run over our prefrontal cortex's rational* desire for cognitive reasoning and response with a hypersensitive immediate response. Bang![78]

The amygdala jumps first and thinks later. Too often, the amygdala wins, controlling our responses. The prefrontal cortex is no match for your amygdala once it's triggered.

Once out of the gate, it becomes a problematic steed to pull back. It will take twenty minutes to settle down after a blowup. Perhaps you'll convince yourself of the righteousness of your indignation or ignore and forget about the incident altogether.[79] Rational brain is left to pick up the pieces almost while the emotional brain hides.

Anger is good when properly activated, destructive, and unhealthy when uncontrolled. The same concept applies to fear. In its proper function, fear alerts us to potential harm. Unbridled fear imagines situations that either don't exist or become highly exaggerated. Living in uncontrolled fear freezes many lives from reaching their full potential.

Anger's Effects On Mental Health

In *Depression is More Than Just Sadness: A Case of Excessive Anger and Its Management in Depression*, Anamika Sahu Preeti Gupta, and Biswadip Chatterjee noted:

People with depressive illness often have symptoms of overt or suppressed anger. Those with anger traits face exaggerated problem during symptomatic period of depression. Pharmacological management helps in control of depressive and anxiety symptoms, but rarely address anger symptoms.[80]

Many studies link anger and depression.[81] Up to ninety percent of nonclinical depression is linked to anger.[82] Anger and depression often coexist.

The *American Addictions Centers Resource*, notes;

Anger is both a physiological (body) and psychological (mind) process. Because of this, anger can have a negative impact on your physical and your emotional health. This is particularly true of the relationship between anger and heart disease.[83]

Anger is a Secondary Emotion

Anger always has a root, a catalyst that initiates it. You may tell yourself after an eruption, "Well, it just happened." That's rarely the case. Yes, there are some instances where anger is beyond one's control. A malfunction in the brain, perhaps. However, most of us can anger, but it's a learned skill.

103

"I couldn't help it."

True, if unchecked, until it's too late when anger exceeds our rational ability to throttle back our fury. That's why anger's control must occur early before reaching critical mass. Anger is also an emotion. Emotions in themselves do not think. They're not rational. Ever hear someone say, "I don't know what made me do that?"

Uncontrolled anger becomes an emotional reaction. Only after an angry eruption can the neocortex ask, "What happened?" Then comes dealing with the carnage and wreckage left in anger's wake.

Learning to control the brain before it reacts is imperative.

When anger becomes the fruit falling from our rage trees, it usually points to something bigger than anger's immediate response. That's because anger needs a triggering point to set it off.

What Makes Us So Angry?

In my late teens, my mother worked at Howie's Bar on West Broadway in Minneapolis, Minnesota. Was she a cook, server, or bartender? In part, but believe it or not, my mother was also a bouncer. You know, one of those strong-armed people that eject unruly customers—86ed them—out into the street.

Toward the end of Christmas vacation, it was time to begin the eight-hour drive to Bible College, where I was preparing for ministry. My goodbyes would occur in a pub, or beer joint, as it was called in our local dialect.

As I came around a corner on a frigid, icy day, a man screamed obscenities at his car. In the below-zero weather, the car wouldn't start. The more he tried to start his car, the angrier he grew as the groaning engine failed to fire. Then he opened the trunk and pulled out a shovel. Hurling obscenities, he shattered every window of his car. By the time he finished his tirade, the vehicle was wrecked. With that, he collapsed into a drunken state onto the curb.

As I entered the bar to see my mother, everyone stood looking through the window at the fury that had just finished taking place. One guy asked another, "What made him do that?"

The man reentered the bar in his drunken stupor, unknowingly answering the patron's question, "Nothing ever works out for me! Nothing!"

Unmet needs often trigger anger. We need love, respect, and care. When needs go unmet, especially during child development, it provides a catalyst for seething anger.[84]

Your spouse doesn't respond in a desired manner: anger.
You don't get that promotion: anger.
Someone ignores you: anger.
Anger is often our conditioned go-to response.

Anger can also result from learned behavior. My parents modeled anger repeatedly. Looking back, I now see many of their unmet needs. As a young child, I could not interpret my parents' angry emotions. I only feared them. Sometimes, anger comes from another's influence. It reflects the effects of others on us. Anger becomes a conditioned response when repeatedly modeled by others who influence us. It develops into a go-to reaction.

Hurt inflicted upon us by others is also a significant trigger source. I see this in our adopted grandchildren. They suffered immensely during their early years of development before being removed from their environments. As the saying goes, 'Hurt people, hurt people.' This, sadly, often is true.

Missed expectations become a weighty source of anger. Missionaries constantly share their disappointments when resigning from fields of service. "It wasn't what I thought it would be," they cry.

One pastor said, "Wow, this is nothing like they told me it would be during the interview process. I thought I could make friends here."

There's the marriage, "My spouse became a different person."

At work, "That's not a part of my job description."

Or, "I thought I could win."

And, "This is so different from what I thought it was going to be like."

Explicit expectations become precise in our minds. What are you looking for in a job, relationship, church, doctor, and so on? The problem is with every expectation, scores of implicit anticipations follow. Things you believe everyone else sees and knows like you do.[85]

Uncontrolled anger is possibly the most damaging of all emotions.

When expectations go unfulfilled, for some, an emotional simmering begins. Then anger spews out like a volcano or withdraws and hides.

Trying to protect ourselves, we often hurt those around us. Anger can protect us, but uncontrolled, it's probably the most damaging of all emotions, springing out of unmet needs, unfulfilled expectations, or insecurities.[86]

Find anger's source. Without discovering, acknowledging, and managing its root cause, anger dangles us like marionette puppets powerless to control.

Bitterness: A Real Culprit Too

While unmet needs, hurt, failed expectations, and insecurities lead to anger, *I credit some of our anger to bitterness.*[87] Some might argue this as mere semantics, but bitterness stands on its own here.

Bitterness is resentment towards someone, an event, misfortune, or station in life that we couldn't control to our satisfaction.

In its root element, anger's source is bitterness. Bitterness stems from resentment at what I couldn't control.

That's why Dr. Luke the Apostle warned:

Work at living in peace with everyone, and work at living a holy life, for those who are not holy will not see the Lord. Look after each other so that none of you fails to receive the grace of God. **Watch out that no poisonous root of bitterness grows** up to trouble you, corrupting many.

Hebrews 12:14-15 Emphasis Mine

Paul shows a clear connection between bitterness and severe anger:

Get rid of **all bitterness**, **rage**, **anger**, **harsh words**, and **slander**, as well as all types of evil behavior. Ephesians 4:31

Note the progression:

Bitterness – a bitter root producing angry, pungent, resentful fruit.[88]

Rage – fiery anger, passion.[89]

Anger – violent emotion.[90]

Harsh Words – verbal lashings that wound and destroy.

Slander – from the word *blasphemia,* from which our word 'blasphemy' is derived. Meaning to speak injury to another's good name. To tarnish a person's character. Damage their reputation.[91]

Bitterness can come in many forms. Failure to be treated respectfully. A letdown of a trusted family member. Disappointment with the agency you work for. A sense of not being treated the way you should be treated. Something withheld that you believe you deserve. *Bitterness stems from resentment at being unable to get what is thought to be owed.*

> *Look deep into your anger. Often, bitterness lies at its source.*

I find a good question to ask: "What makes me so resentful about this?"

Getting Your Anger Under Control

Missionary, pastor, Christian, deal with your anger before it ruins you, others, and everything around you.

I talk about missionaries because I've spent thirty years as a missionary. Currently, Kathy and I serve missionaries again. From many sessions spent with missionaries, I can tell you we harbor unhealthy levels of bitterness.

Pastors, we're no better. As a young traveling missionary in the 1980s, I often stopped at a local breakfast café in Wichita, Kansas. A half dozen pastors in their fifties and sixties met for coffee every week. I quite enjoyed dropping in on those meetings.

Six years later, after returning from my first term in South Africa, I stopped at that same café. That morning, only one pastor sat at a table. It didn't take long for him to tell the story.

An argument broke out between those pastors two years prior. The rancor grew until they refused to see each other again. Once like-minded, now they repudiated each other. The sad part? Most of them died refusing to speak with one another again.

James, the brother of Jesus, had something to say about all this:

Understand this, my dear brothers and sisters: You must all be *quick to listen*, *slow* *to speak*, and *slow* *to get angry. Human anger does not produce the righteousness God desires.*

James 1:19-20 Italics Mine

'Slow' is an interesting word James uses here. It's the Koine Greek word *bradys* used only three times in the entire New Testament, two times in this verse alone. The word implies being dense, stupid, inactive, or slow to apprehend.

The only other time it's used outside this verse is when Jesus reprimanded the travelers on the road to Emmaus:

Then he said unto them, O fools, and *slow* of heart to believe all that the prophets have spoken.

Luke 24:25 KJV Emphasis Mine

What's James saying about anger? *Let us be dense and slow to apprehend anger.* Seems people back then struggled with anger, too.

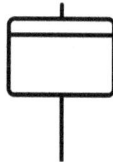

Controlling Your Anger

James Three Laws of Anger Control

Law # 1 Open Your Ears!

"You all must be quick to listen..." James 1:19

I like St. Francis of Assisi's Peace Prayer:

Lord, make me an instrument of your peace:
where there is hatred, let me sow love;
where there is injury, pardon;
where there is doubt, faith;
where there is despair, hope;
where there is darkness, light;
where there is sadness, joy.
O divine Master, *grant that I may not so much seek*
to be consoled as to console,
to be understood as to understand,
to be loved as to love.
For it is in giving that we receive,
it is in pardoning that we are pardoned,
and it is in dying that we are born to eternal life. Amen.

Law #2 Shut Your Mouth

"Let every person be slow to speak." James 1:19

When anger churns, learn the discipline of remaining silent. Never speak in anger. Most times, words clouded in anger hurl injurious misjudgments. How often have you blown up, stoked up, or seeped out putrefied emotions only to discover that you misunderstood the situation? That's if we're honest and brave enough to examine what caused our anger.

This one principle could help you conquer your anger. *Close your mouth until your anger calms down.*

Don't fire that email off.

Don't make that phone call.

Don't post your anger on social media.

Don't respond sarcastically. Sarcasm often stems from anger.

Don't respond until you're rational.

Law #3 Slow Your Anger

"… slow to get angry." James 1:19

Stupefy your anger. Deactivate it. Depower it. Tell it, "You don't have the right to speak here. Maybe later, but not right now." Note three alternatives offered to anger in Ephesians:

Get rid of all bitterness, rage, anger, harsh words, and slander, as well as all types of evil behavior. Instead, [1]**be kind** to each other, [2]**tenderhearted,** [3] **forgiving one another**, just as God through Christ has forgiven you. Ephesians 4:31-32

The Anger Control Formula

Instead:

[1]**Replace anger with kindness**. Mild and pleasant—as opposed to harsh, sharp, and bitter.[92] Replace anger with another emotion. Rather than becoming harsh, become gentle. Put a smile over a grimacing face. Calmness rather than aggressiveness.

[2] **Respond tenderheartedly**. This word used for 'tenderhearted' in Ephesians 4:31-32 means 'having strong bowels.' Hold your anger. Wait for an appropriate moment to release it. [93] Get the idea?

³ **Instead of ill temper, choose forgiveness**. How much forgiveness? What kind of forgiveness? "… forgiving one another just as God through Christ has forgiven you."

The qualifier is, how much did God forgive you? Match your forgiveness for others with God's forgiveness of you. Forgiveness acted upon deactivates anger.

RAAD

This little acrostic I developed helps me stay out of trouble. Maybe it'll help you, too. R.A.A.D. stands for:

Recognize when you're angry.

Acknowledge anger's source.

Access a plan to deal with your anger.

Decide on your course of action and stick with it.

Practicing R.A.A.D can become a valuable tool in dealing with your anger.

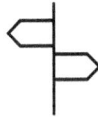

Other considerations

Chip Ingram and Dr. Becca Johnson encourage an excellent strategy for dealing with anger: [94]

1. **Minimize Stress**.
   Get rid of what you don't need.
   Become a minimalist.

Let some things go.

Chip declares, "The more pressured, burned out, overwhelmed, or busy we are, the more vulnerable we are to anger."

2. **Maximize God**. Again, James gives us very helpful advice here:

Come close to God, and God will come close to you. Wash your hands, you sinners; purify your hearts, for your loyalty is divided between God and the world. James 4:8

Get close to God. Pull close to your Creator when tempted by anger. This becomes a rational function of the brain. Besides its spiritual impact, focusing upon God kicks the prefrontal cortex into action, controlling the limbic system's sometimes irrational responses.

Come close to God, and God **will come close to you**.

James 4:8

Remember, anger is your responsibility. Own it. Deal with it. Make amends to others you've hurt with it. Most of all, learn to live above your anger.

People with understanding control their anger; a *hot temper shows* great *foolishness*.

Proverbs 14:29 Emphasis Mine

Other Resources to Help You Deal with Your Anger

Chip Ingram, in his series *Relationships Under Pressure* and the book *Overcoming Emotions that Destroy: Practical Help for Those Angry Feelings That Ruin Relationships*, talks about three faces of anger.

Also, get a hold of Chip's podcast: *Relationships Under Pressure: Keeping it Together When the World's Falling Apart.*
https://livingontheedge.org/broadcast-series/relationships-under-pressure/

Bilodeau, L. (1997). *The anger workbook.* MJF Books.

Ingram, C. (2013). *Overcoming emotions that destroy: practical help for those angry feelings that ruin relationships: small group study guide.* Living on the edge with Chip Ingram.

Jackson, T. (1994). *When anger burns.* Radio Bible Class.

Jones, R. D. (2005). *Uprooting anger: biblical help for a common problem.* P & R Publications.

Mack, W. A. (2017*). Anger and Stress Management God's Way.* P & R Publishing.

McKay, M., Rogers, P. D., & McKay, J. (2003). *When anger hurts: quieting the storm within.* New Harbinger Publications.

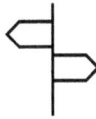

Anger's Powerful Ally: Bitterness

We've already talked a bit about how bitterness plays a part in our angry responses. Let's delve deeper.

As bitterness slowly permeates us, it pollutes the soul's core. It's sort of like a leaking septic system. As raw sewage leaks into the groundwater, it contaminates the drinking water coming up from a well. So, too, does bitterness. It leaks into every ounce of our being, poisoning ourselves and those around us.

Question: Is bitterness leaking from your soul?

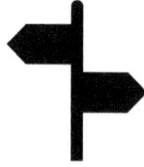

Guidepost #9
Bitter Attitudes Leak

Look after each other so that none of you fails to receive the grace of God. Watch out that no poisonous root of bitterness grows up to trouble you, corrupting many.

Hebrews 12:15

"Nothing consumes a man more quickly than the emotion of resentment."

Friedrich Nietzsche

EVERY SUMMER AS A KID, my grandparents took our family to great-grandpa and grandma's cabin! The cabin sat on a channel connecting Roosevelt and Lawrence Lake in Northern Minnesota. Splendid memories flood my mind of those pleasant summer experiences. But a few not-so-great recollections remain, too.

The cabin's drinking water came from a well through a pipe that went down into the ground. The hum of the electric motor pulling water up from the well into the faucets of the cabin reminded us we'd arrived at the lake.

Now, the water was perfectly healthy to drink. But in those early days, the water carried a high mineral content before Grandpa punched a new well. It tasted awful. The metallic concoction of iron, zinc, and copper lingered long after we swallowed it. Grandpa had the water tested. Besides the taste, it was healthy to drink. My younger brother once commented that the water at the cabin tasted like drinking pennies.

Yet that 'perfectly healthy' water carried consequences. Unaccustomed to the cabin water, our juvenile stomachs struggled to process it. This filled the septic tank to the brim, causing unpleasant reverberations. Doses of Pepto-Bismol, a pink chalky go-to mint potion of the day, failed to mitigate the strain on our tummies, nor the overflowing septic tank.

Mom always tried to mask the metallurgic taste with a unique cocktail. In those days, Kool-Aid was only available unsweetened in small packets. Grape-flavored Kool-Aid proved most efficient at hiding the unwanted tang.

The directions read, "One packet per gallon." So, mom tore open two small packets, emptying them into a gallon plastic pitcher. Along with that came twice the recommended dosage of sugar; four heaping cups, as I remember. Filling the jug with water from the tap, we took turns stirring the flavorful sludge at the bottom.

Then came the coup de grâce as mom added four small, sliced lemon wedges into the mix to slay the bitter-salty taste. A couple of trays of ice tossed in, and voila!

Yet, the water still tasted like those copper pennies prevalent in the 1960s. Its bitterness left an aftertaste difficult to mask.

Like the water at my great-grandparent's cabin, high bitterness content in our attitudes leaves unpleasant aftereffects. Bitterness taints us, leaving those around us affected as well.

The Bitterness Plague

Bitterness has continually plagued Christians since the beginning of the Church. Bitterness is rarely self-contained and poisons our thinking, spilling out onto others.

Sometimes bitterness results from the grind of life. Slogging it out. Seeing little return for your labors. Haven't we all been there? As life wears us down, our outlook turns sour. A disdain towards others faring better than ourselves can cloud relationships.

For others, resentment develops from past wounds. The injustices of life. Mistreatment from others. Living with a long-term disease or disability. Losing your family when another nation invades your homeland. Economic disparity. Social injustices. And… for many, once employed by the church, resentment at being used, disrespected, or discarded.

Behind many successful churches lie the bones of those who helped garner a church's success. Many previous staff members or volunteers feel justified in their bitterness because of perceived mistreatment from 'spiritual leaders.'

Missionaries who believe Christians let them down.

Pastors, who are mistreated by a vocal minority of ecclesiastical terrorists within their church, lose hope in the very place, claiming to offer hope.

People who 'used to go to church' but refuse to enter the church again, citing an episode or exchange that didn't favor them.

People who 'used to go to church,' but refuse to enter the church again, citing an episode or exchange that didn't favor them.

Sometimes, bitterness appears justified. Perhaps it is. Life is unfair. People are cruel. Within every church sits fallen, frail, sinful beings who fail to treat others as Paul admonished, "In humility, value others above yourselves." Philippians 2:3-4

While it may feel justified, bitterness possesses zero benefits. Its negative pull forces a mental tug of war-with our thinking and emotions. It damages our relationship with God, others, and ourselves.

Too often in the church, I've watched bitterness develop over nothing and everything. And resentment usually attracts allies, providing a rallying point for shared consumption of its venom.

The Church-kitchen Wars

Once, the kitchen of our church became a war zone. One volunteer got upset that people entered the kitchen to get a cup of coffee before the set 9:15 coffeetime on Sunday morning.

And EVERYONE knows that when Moses came down from the mount with the two tablets, the eleventh command read, "Thou shalt not enter the kitchen before 9:15 coffeetime."

Others on the 'coffee team' complained. Before you knew it, ten volunteers over five different Sundays—two volunteers to a Sunday—began castigating anyone even nearing the kitchen before 9:15.

No one appreciates the work we do here in the kitchen!
People take us for granted!
And our pastor doesn't care either.
Those people don't deserve coffee!

Volunteers making the coffee augured the need for boundaries. Church members entered the kitchen, claiming it was their 'right' to do so. The rancor had raged for years before becoming their pastor. Sure, each side carried legitimate grievances, but neither capitulated to the other. They refused to follow Christ's example in serving each other. Bitterness ruled.

Don't look out only for your own interests, but take an interest in others, too. You must have the same attitude that Christ Jesus had.

Philippians 2: 4-5

One particular Sunday, a visitor sat in the gym with a hundred other people outside the closed, rolling counter door at the kitchen service window. Looking for the bathroom, she entered one of the side doors into the kitchen and suffered a blistering rebuke.

She never returned to the church whose mantra was *Loving God, Loving People.*

Those sullied attitudes far exceeded the bitterness of that cheap, crummy coffee brewed in the kitchen.

I settled the issue. Arriving on Sunday morning at 6:00 AM, the church always stood dark and empty. My first destination became the kitchen.

When people entered a few hours later, two 100-cup coffee pots stood ready to dispense freshly brewed coffee on a table in the gymnasium outside the kitchen. All the condiments for coffee time lay on the table, too. Members commented on how wonderful the church smelled as the coffee's scent filled the lobby.

While I never let on who made the coffee every Sunday morning, someone figured it out. After that, volunteers began arriving at 7:30 to make coffee for ANYONE AT ANYTIME wanting a cup of coffee.

My First Church Business Meeting

At my first church business meeting, 'born-again Bible-believing Christians' effortlessly modeled bitterness. There, someone erupted about a past issue. I was sixteen, and don't remember what the matter was, but demarcated groups went to war on the floor of that 'holy' sanctuary.

One ringleader yelled accusations at the pastor, demanding people leave the church. Found out later that the screaming fellow was also involved in a sexual affair with another woman.

Now, as mentioned, my mother worked as a bouncer at Howie's Bar in North Minneapolis, Minnesota, when I was a kid. Mom's world of profanity and edginess never really bothered me much. In verbal contests among inebriated patrons, they often mentioned god. Deity saturated most of the yelling matches and fistfights, too.

Now, the 'godly' people in the business meeting that night at church never used a foul word like those drunk sods in the bar where my mother worked. They did, however, use the word 'God' a lot. 'God' became their weapon of choice. With it, they slayed those around them.

Looking back, it's not surprising that the church closed its doors a few years later. The world doesn't need a church like that, anyway. No one does.

> *Bitterness often is a meal of self-devourment.*

Bitterness triggers destructive behaviors. In the end, bitterness is a meal of self-devourment, dealing self-inflicted wounds to the carrier rather than a perceived enemy. It's also often a major component of mental health. Many dealing with mental health challenges cite injustices of the past that they cannot overlook. The more they speak of an incident, the angrier or more anxious they become. The sullying of their person because someone did them wrong.

A betrayal.

Victimization.

That insult.

Broken promise.

A lie.

Injury by someone once trusted.

Something that they can't get over.

Do any of these apply to you? How long ago did bitterness wrap its tentacles around you, squeezing potential goodness and happiness from your heart? What exactly is it that leaves you unable to uncover the object of your bitterness?

I've listened to many cross-cultural workers and pastors whose bitterness often boiled down to a deep-seated resentment towards God more than people. *An inability to control circumstances towards a preferred desirable outcome, which they believe God abandoned them.*

120

Bitterness and Mental Health

Members in the two churches I pastored in Minnesota frequently came to me for council. A few wanted someone to justify their bitterness, reinforcing their hostility towards others.

Without exception, every person I've ever known who's dwelt in long seasons of bitterness also suffered from mental health issues. That's not to say every person struggling with mental health is bitter. Yet, it's tragically fascinating that bitter people often carry destructive seeds within their mental DNA.

Dr. Stephen A. Diamond in *Psychology Today* tries to tackle this:

Most mental disorders stem either directly from—or secondarily generate—anger, rage, resentment, hostility or bitterness. [95]

He adds:

Bitterness, which I define as a chronic and pervasive state of *smoldering resentment*, is one of the most destructive and toxic of human emotions. Bitterness is a kind of morbid characterological hostility toward someone, something or toward life itself, resulting from the consistent repression of anger, rage or resentment regarding how one really has or perceives to have been treated. Bitterness is a prolonged, resentful feeling of disempowered and devalued victimization. *Embitterment, like resentment and hostility, results from the long-term mismanagement* of annoyance, irritation, frustration, anger or rage. [96] Italics mine.

The Bible and Bitterness

Dr. Luke warned us:

Look after each other so that none of you fails to receive the grace of God. Watch out that *no poisonous root of bitterness grows up* to trouble you, **corrupting** many.

Hebrews 12:15 Emphasis Mine

Corrupting, a very descriptive word. In other versions of the Bible, it's translated from the Hebrew word *miainō* as 'defiled' or 'troubles.' Homer's Iliad uses a synonym of *miainō*.

In Scroll 4, line 141 it begins, "As when some woman of Meonia or Caria strains **purple dye** on to a piece of ivory…"[97]

The word used by Homer is "to dye with another color, or to stain." [98]

Miainō used in the Book of Hebrews implies "defilement because of an action." [99] A discoloration of a person through bitter reasoning.

Choosing bitterness degrades our relationships with God, others, and ourselves. Bitterness stains us, turning us—dyeing us—into something else.

Josephus, the Roman historian during the writings of the books of the New Testament, used this same word. This word common in his writings carried the idea of "cultic pollution." [100]

Bitterness: a cultic pollution, creating unreasonable zealots. A disposition that produces unreasonable, irrational people. That pegs what I've witnessed in myself and others in every church I've pastored.

The Bible recognizes that prolonged bitterness carries detrimental effects. It affects not only our mental health but our entire well-being. So, if bitterness is so damaging, what makes it so prevalent in our lives?

The Source of Bitterness

Dr. J. Ryan Fuller—a clinical psychologist—notes:

… researchers found, first of all, that **bitterness** is most likely to stem from failure at something. Another finding was that anger and accusation usually accompany **bitterness**, indicating that it is different from regret, where any anger or blame is turned inward on oneself. The bitter person aims his anger, hostility, and blame at someone or something else. Whenever you fail at what you're trying to accomplish, do you tend to blame yourself or others (e.g., teacher, spouse, boss, government).[101] Emphasis Mine

The source of bitterness is often the person themselves:

I'd be okay if it had worked out this way or that way.
They laid me off from my job.
The church fired me for no good reason.
My missions agency called us home.
The church wanted to get rid of me.
He left me.
She left me.
My father abandoned me.
Mom ran out on us.
Because of that I...

> *Bitterness often boils down to selfishness. A focus on what I want or think I deserve.*

And God often gets the blame for our misfortunes. Resentment germinates because the Creator doesn't comply with our wishes. Then, we validate our tarnished attitudes toward people and life with the following:

Yes, but you don't understand how much that person hurt me.
What they did to me.
How they lied to me.
What they cost me financially.
How unfair it is.
Why is it so unforgivable?

True. I'm not negating the pain or its adverse effects. But bitterness makes everything worse. Simple as that.

Bitterness becomes easily justifiable.

A dislike of another person.

Verbal barrages to vilify another.

Hatred towards an establishment or company.

Despising an entire people group.

Could the source of your bitterness be you?

Loathing all churches because of one's actions.

Hating all men because a man hurt you.

Hostility towards all women because of the treatment received from your mother, wife, girlfriend, or boss.

A cynical incapacity to trust another missionary because a missionary mistreated you.

Or, as with current revelations, all clergy are predators because of the few lowlifes discovered using their authority and position to take advantage of others, often young children.

Bitterness often provokes an easy, although damaging, response. Most times, bitterness is a sin. Yet, in some situations, bitterness seems a mechanism of coping with egregious hurts and trauma forced upon us.

I think, however, the primary reason the Bible instructs us to get rid of all bitterness is because of its devastating power in our lives. Bitterness ruins and destroys us. It hurts the bitterness-bearer more than anyone else. That's why the Bible encourages:

Get rid of all **bitterness**, rage, anger, harsh words, and slander, as well as all types of evil behavior.

Ephesians 4:31

Bitterness: A lack of trust in God

Bitterness can frequently boil down to resentment and a lack of trust in God. Paul's words here in Romans 8:28 are hard for us to swallow. It reminds us that what happens to and around us far exceeds our ability to see the entire picture.

And we know that *God causes everything to work together* for the good of those who love God and are called according to his purpose for them.

We understand only a shadow of what happens to us. Only God sees the entire picture, working all things towards a cumulative goal. That's why I'm learning to ask different questions.

Instead of *"Why?"* I try to ask God, *"What and How?"*

God, what are you doing here?
What's working together towards a good cause?
What is a suitable response?
What should I do here?
How do you desire me to become more like your son, Jesus Christ?

Becoming more like Jesus is the goal of the happenings in our lives. "For God knew his people in advance, and he chose them to become like his Son..." Romans 8:29a

If we can see our Creator bringing all things together—even though we don't understand—then releasing resentment and bitterness becomes possible. All the goings-on in our lives ultimately come together towards a meaningful purpose. Can you trust God with this?

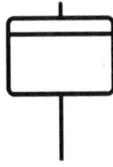

Personal Prayer: An Effective Weapon Against Bitterness

A Personal Prayer

God, hear me and answer me.

You know I am troubled by thoughts and feelings of anger, resentment, and bitterness.

You also know why. And You know how deep my hurt goes and how long I have lived with it.

But I don't want to live with bitterness any longer. I don't want to be an angry, resentful person.

With Your help, I release my anger into Your hands. I surrender my resentment. I let go of my bitterness.

Help me keep letting go, releasing toxic emotions when they try to arise.[102]

Amen

My Prayer Mentor

Our Father, Who art in heaven, hallowed be Thy name;
Thy kingdom come;
Thy will be done on earth as it is in heaven.
Give us this day our daily bread;
and *forgive* us our trespasses *as we forgive* those who trespass against us;
and lead us not into temptation, but deliver us from evil.

☐ Jesus

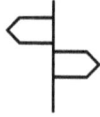

A Prayer to Ponder

Let me learn to focus first upon you, Lord,
    then upon others,
        and only then upon myself.
Let my soul look to you when I'm in pain.
    When in unbelief,
        as I question your presence, may I trust that you're where
            I think you're not.
When I complain,
    help me look and smile towards you.
Rather than putting myself in the center of me,
    let me center myself in you.
Help me celebrate what I'm able to do
    rather than grieve that which I've lost the ability to perform.
And every day,
    remind me of something for which I can be thankful,
        you've surrounded me with good people and things.

Amen.

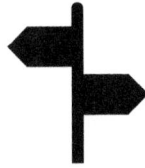

Guidepost #10

Social Media — Not Always Social

BEFORE YOU WRITE ME OFF as an old sod who constantly carps about the evils of social media, let me assure you that the opposite is true.

Currently, I sport two X accounts, several Facebook pages, a LinkedIn page, two Instagrams, and a Reddit account. Social media, for me, is a valuable tool for communicating with family, missionaries, pastors, and friends. These SNSs—social networking services—also help supporters stay current on our efforts to serve missionaries.

It's also the primary mode of keeping up with our sixteen grandchildren. Seeing pictures and videos of them keeps us connected with their special moments of life.

I love my social media!

Yet, there is a lot of information out there on the damaging effects of SNSs on our mental health, too.

I'm not encouraging you to get rid of all your social media. What I am saying is to learn to control your Social Media. *Balance is the key.*

A Personal View

Before SNSs, our social networking comprised the telephone, video, and cassette tapes sent through the postal system, along with stamped letters and packages. As the 90s rolled around, we began using services like AOL, CompuServe, Prodigy or Ask Jeeves.

Many of us breeze in and out of the cyberworld, social media making up much of the time spent there. Much of social media, TikTok, Facebook, Instagram, YouTube, and WhatsApp, just to name a few, does not reflect real life.

Disclaimer here, I've used every app just listed.

Now, I'm not saying give up your social media. Nor am I failing to acknowledge the benefits of social media.

During the Covid-19 crisis, SNSs provided valuable tools to communicate around the world. I can't remember how many Zoom sessions, Facebook chats, and other social medias occurred with missionaries worldwide.

So, let's use the myriads of tools at our disposal today. Learn to increase your effectiveness in communicating God's love to the nations. Stay in touch with your friends and families.

Ease the tension with a game or two. I love Last War. It's a complex game with 100s of moving pieces. In my alliance, I intermingle with Professors, Doctors, Engineers, and business owners, just to name a few.

Use social media as a tool towards better health. On Facebook, I belong to several groups. One is Living with FSHD. In this group, those who suffer with FSHD Muscular Dystrophy, like myself, discuss many facets of living and dealing with this debilitating disease.

So, use social media and enjoy it, but don't let your media become an idol. Your supreme consideration upon waking up, constantly checking your phone throughout the day and fixating upon it before sleeping.

Also, don't allow it to become a source of sin. You know what I'm saying. There's an abundance of toxic trash in the cyberworld. Be careful, my friend, for many ruined lives lie in the internet's cesspools.

And don't put too much emphasis upon the 'likes.' We all like likes. Right? Remember that our lives are not about likes. They're about following Jesus.

Psychological Implications to Mental Health

McClean Hospital, a Harvard Medical School Associate, published in an article, *The Social Dilemma: Social Media and Your Mental Health*:

> 'Like' it or not, using social media can cause anxiety, depression, and other health challenges… Social media has a reinforcing nature. Using it activates the brain's reward center by releasing dopamine, a "feel-good chemical" linked to pleasurable activities such as sex, food, and social interaction. The platforms are designed to be addictive and are associated with anxiety, depression, and even physical ailments.[103]

The National Center for Health Research asserts:

> Many studies have found an association between time spent on social media as well as the number of social media platforms used, and symptoms of depression and anxiety… in one study from 2020, people who deactivated their Facebook account for a month reported lower depression and anxiety, as well as increases in happiness and life satisfaction.[104]

Depression, Anxiety Disorders, and Social Media

A study from the *Journal of Affective Disorders* asserts, "… that more daily social media use was significantly associated with a greater likelihood of a probable anxiety disorder,"[105]

Help Guide, lists five negative effects from overexposure to social media:

- Inadequacy about your life or appearance.
- Fear of missing out (FOMO) and social media addiction.
- Isolation,
- Depression and anxiety.
- Cyber-bullying.
- Self-absorption.[106]

Mental Health America asserts, "Even before COVID-19, the prevalence of mental illness among adults was increasing. In 2017-2018, 19% of adults experienced a mental illness, an increase of 1.5 million people over last year's dataset." [107]

> *Don't put too much emphasis on 'likes.'*

Some disagree. One point is certain, mental health issues continue to rise among all population groups. Pastors, missionaries, and Christians are not exempt.

Try to make your social media a positive experience. Use the connective tools social media provides. Just be careful. That's all I'm saying.

Don't allow social media's temptations to snag your mental and spiritual vitality, putting it above your walk and worship of our Lord.

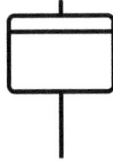

When in Doubt...

Philippians 4:8 offers us the best guide when interacting on social media and SNSs:

> And now, dear brothers and sisters, one final thing. Fix your thoughts on what is true, and honorable, and right, and pure, and lovely, and admirable. *Think about things that are excellent and worthy of praise.*

Fix your thoughts – the idea is to dwell, move in, and make your thinking or your mental health live within boundaries.[108]

What is true – literally, 'thoughts that are not concealed.' A truth that is something that can be trusted.

And, how much on the internet can actually be trusted?[109]

Honorable – the Greek root for this word is *sebo*. It carries the idea of revering or worshipping. Ask yourself this question when on social media, "What is the object of my worship?"[110]

Scrolling endlessly on the internet wastes our lives, doing nothing except filling our minds with images and information that overload our mental capacities to think.

How about Fantasy Football? Whew! I'm touching the holy grail now. I'm in a fantasy football league with my family. However, it must not consume me.

Now, we have online gambling. Remember, it takes a thousand people losing money for one person to win. Reminds me of an old saying, "To gamble and lose is foolish, but to gamble and win is theft."

Ask yourself when on the internet, "What am I worshipping here?"

Right – that which is virtuous, innocent, guiltless, or righteous.[111]

Pure – that which is pure from carnality, modest, and faultless. Well, that eliminates much of what social media offers. Doesn't it?[112]

Lovely – that which is acceptable, pleasing, or friendly towards.[113]

Admirable – that which is of good repute. Things spoken kindly with goodwill towards others.[114]

Philippians 4:8 offers us a flawless guide to social media exposure. It's up to us to put these principles into practice.

This verse finishes with,

> *"Think about things that are excellent and worthy of praise."*

Excellence, of high value. Praise that which is worth commendation, appreciation, or accolades.[115]

Applying this to our social media use, balance will follow.

Balance is the key.

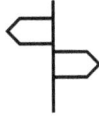

Controlling Your Social Media Exposure

Suggestions

- Spend more time with your offline friends.
- Use an app tracker to see how much time you spend on social media.
- Take a social media break.
- Schedule a 'phone turn off' time every day.
- Disable those social media alerts! You don't need the constant pestering of a buzzing, beeping phone all day.
- Reduce your social media apps.
- Limit the amount of times you check your phone during the day.
- How about a 'smartphone' free day zone? No phone for an entire day.[116]

Website Tools

www.xxxchurch.com offers tremendous helps for controlling media exposure.

www.covenanteyes.com is another excellent source of internet control and spiritual encouragement.

www.connectsafely.org/parents-guide-to-tiktok helps you control children's exposure to TikTok.

You can also use the **Restricted Mode** on TikTok to help control what you see as well. Although, after investigating this, it's not foolproof.

www.keyhole.co/blog/social-media-monitoring-tools offers many sites for social monitoring tools.

www.accountable2you.com offers an internet filter to block dangerous or inappropriate websites.

www.everaccountable.com filters porn sites and other dangers on the internet.

Remember

> Pure and undefiled religion before God and the Father is this… **to keep oneself unspotted from the world.**

James 1:27

Part IV

Positive Mental Health Practices

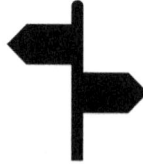

Guidepost #11

Spiritual Mindfulness
Minds the Mind

You will keep in perfect peace
all who trust in you,
all whose thoughts are fixed on you!

Isaiah 26:3

MINDFULNESS IS A COMMON TOPIC these days. Often, it's taught as a meditative guide to become fully aware of what you're sensing in the moment without interpretation or judgment of the event.[117] That's not where we're going here.

This loosely defined concept that has gained popularity exists in all the major religions of the world.[118] The writers of the Bible long ago cited the importance of spiritual mindfulness, a quieting of our person for a specific purpose. Asaph declared, Asaph declared,

I remember the days of old. I ponder all your great works and think about what you have done. I lift my hands to you in prayer. I thirst for you as parched land thirsts for rain. Psalms 77:5-6

What is Spiritual Mindfulness?

Generally, mindfulness is learning to focus deliberately on the present without allowing other thoughts to continually run through your head. It's a clearing of the noise from your mind.[119]

Again, the Bible had this figured out centuries ago:

I have calmed and quieted myself, like a weaned child who no longer cries for its mother's milk. Yes, like a weaned child is my soul within me.

Psalm 131:2

Spiritual Mindfulness concentrates on God in me and me in God. A sensing of being with God in each moment while interacting with myself and ourselves.[120] In sense God's presence throughout the day, we can become much more understanding of our thoughts, actions, and words. It is a practice needing development for good mental and spiritual health.

The Psalm writer talked about this:

But they delight in the law of the Lord, **meditating** on it day and night."

Psalm 1:2 Emphasis Mine

In the busy Evangelical culture of the West, we often measure God's relationships through our religious activities. Attending church functions, musical worship concerts, meetings, small groups, generosity, and other doings mark our mindfulness. What we do for God often parallels our understanding of Emmanuel, God with us.

Dynamics of Spiritual Mindfulness

Spiritual mindfulness centers upon several aspects of Christ's teachings in the Sermon on the Mount:

1. Life is more important than our basic desires. Matthew 6:25
2. Worry underestimates our value to God. Matthew 6:26
3. Worry lacks trust in God's promise to provide. Matthew 6:30
4. Worry questions about whether God is fully aware of my needs. Matthew 6:31
5. Worry doubts God's ability to provide for us. Matthew 6:33
6. Worry overwhelms our ability to navigate today's issues. Matthew 6:34

With Christ's words in Matthew Chapter 6, spiritual mindfulness makes God our primary consideration, not ourselves. It pushes God's care for us to the front of our prefrontal cortex, allowing faith and rational thought to control overreactive limbic systems. This helps reduce worry, for example, as trusting God becomes our primary focus.

With Christ's words in Matthew Chapter 6, spiritual mindfulness makes God our primary consideration, not ourselves. It pushes God's care for us to the front of our prefrontal cortex, allowing faith and rational thought to control overreactive limbic systems. This helps reduce worry, for example, as trusting God becomes our primary focus.

We can then ask ourselves, "What's worrying me. What exactly is the issue? What can I do to change the situation? Or how might I learn to trust God in the circumstances facing me?

When we continually worry—sleepless nights, knots in our stomachs, neck pain, digestive problems, pounding heart, panic disorders, phobias, or crushing anxieties—the focus is upon anything else but God.

Spiritual mindfulness simply realizes God's continual presence in our lives. Sounds obvious, right?

Spiritual mindfulness, it's always been a practice of people in the Bible. Consider King David:

> When I look at the night sky and see the work of your fingers—
>   the moon and the stars you set in place—
> what are mere mortals that you should think about them,
>   human beings that you should care for them?
>
> Psalm 8:3-4

Spiritual Mindfulness is a pondering of God's presence in our lives.

> You will keep him in perfect peace, whose mind is stayed on you, because he trusts in You.
>
> Isaiah 26:3 NKJV

Spiritual Christ-centered mindfulness produces Jesus-followers immersed in the Scriptures determined to follow Christ's teachings. The greater our sense of Christ, the more we learn to trust God. "Through Christ you *have come to* trust in God." 1 Peter 1:21 Emphasis Mine

"… have come to…" A maturation process of sensing God's presence in everything. A soundness of mind that should represent every Christ-follower.

> For God has not given us a spirit of fear, but of power and of love and of a sound mind.
>
> 2 Timothy 1:7

Some might argue a misapplication of 2 Timothy 1:7 quoted above, citing that the Greek word *sōphronismos* is often translated as "mind," points towards self-discipline or self-control. No disagreement here. A disciplined life extends from a spiritually fit mind and the will to make it so.

Developing Spiritual Mindfulness

We are instructed and encouraged to develop a spiritually aware mind in many areas:

Mindful of God's presence:

For God has said, "I will never fail you. I will never abandon you.

Deuteronomy 31:6 & Hebrews 13:5

Mindful of Satan's attacks:

Stay alert! Watch out for your great enemy, the devil. He prowls around like a roaring lion, looking for someone to devour.

1 Peter 5:8

Mindful of our bodies:

Don't you realize that your body is the temple of the Holy Spirit, who lives in you and was given to you by God? You do not belong to yourself.

I Corinthians 6:19

Mindful of our relationships with others:

Jesus was aware that his disciples were complaining, so he said to them, "Does this offend you?

141

John 6:61

Soon a Samaritan woman came to draw water, and Jesus said to her, "Please give me a drink." He was alone at the time because his disciples had gone into the village to buy some food.

John 4:7

Someone came to Jesus with this question: 'Teacher, what good deed must I do to have eternal life?' 'Why ask me about what is good?' Jesus replied.

Matthew 19:16-17a

One of the men lying there had been sick for thirty-eight years. When Jesus saw him and knew he had been ill for a long time, he asked him, 'Would you like to get well?'

John 5:5-6

Mindful of surrounding situations:

But the Pharisees went out and conspired against Him, as to how they might destroy Him. But Jesus, aware of this, withdrew from there.

Matthew 12:14-15a NASB

Mindful of grace:

Therefore, with minds that are alert and fully sober, set your hope on the grace to be brought to you when Jesus Christ is revealed at his coming.

1 Peter 1:13 NIV

Mindful of heaven:

Think about the things of heaven, not the things of earth.

Colossians 3:2

Mindful of our spiritual condition:

Those who live according to the flesh have their minds set on what the flesh desires; but those who live in accordance with the Spirit have their minds set on what the Spirit desires. The mind governed by the flesh is death, but the mind governed by the Spirit is life and peace. The mind governed by the flesh is hostile to God; it does not submit to God's law, nor can it do so. Those who are in the realm of the flesh cannot please God.

Romans 8:5-8 NIV

Mindful of our sexuality:

Run from sexual sin! No other sin so clearly affects the body as this one does. For sexual immorality is a sin against your own body. Don't you realize that your body is the temple of the Holy Spirit, who lives in you and was given to you by God? You do not belong to yourself, for God bought you with a high price. So you must honor God with your body.

1 Corinthians 6:18-20

Mindful of fear:

Fear not, for I am with you; Be not dismayed, for I am your God. I will strengthen you, yes, I will help you, I will uphold you with My righteous right hand.

Isaiah 41:10 NKJV

Mindful of depression:

Why, my soul, are you downcast? Why so disturbed within me? Put your hope in God, for I will yet praise him, my Savior and my God.

Psalm 42:11 NIV

143

Mindful of anxiety:

Don't worry about anything; instead, pray about everything. Tell God what you need, and thank him for all he has done. Then you will experience God's peace, which exceeds anything we can understand. His peace will guard your hearts and minds as you live in Christ Jesus.

Philippians 4:6-7

Mindful of perfectionism:

God arms me with strength, and he makes my way perfect.

Psalm 18:32

Mindfulness of self-worth:

If we confess our sins, he is faithful and just to forgive us our sins and to cleanse us from all unrighteousness.

1 John 1:9 ESV

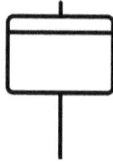

Becoming Mindful

When I am liberated by silence,
when I am no longer involved in the measurement of life,
but in the living of it,
I can discover a form of prayer in which there is
effectively no distraction.
My whole life becomes a prayer.
My whole silence is full of prayer.
The world of silence in which I am immersed contributes
to my prayer.

- Thomas Merton, Life and Holiness

Spiritual mindfulness makes God our primary consideration.

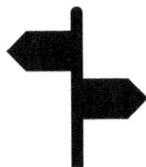

Guidepost #12

Laughter Really is the Best Medicine

IT MIGHT SURPRISE YOU TO know that the above saying, so widely used over the centuries, is almost a direct quote from the Bible:

A cheerful heart is good medicine, but a broken spirit saps a person's strength.

Proverbs 17:22

Over 3,000 years ago, King Solomon advised that laughter is healthy. What modern psychology has recently begun discussing in the last fifty years or so, an ancient king prescribed almost three thousand years ago.

When listening to someone bemoan a situation, and there may be justified reasons for their plight, I like to ask a question. "When was the last time you laughed?"

"Really? What's laughing got to do with it?" Smiles and laughter provide powerful mental health supplements. Well then, when was the last time you laughed?

The Mayo Clinic staff, in an article, *Stress Relief from Laughter? It's No Joke* notes, "Whether you're guffawing at a sitcom on TV or quietly giggling at a newspaper cartoon, laughing does you good. Laughter is a significant form of stress relief, and that's no joke." [121]

Short-term Benefits of Laughter

The Mayo Clinic Staff—no strangers to sad, unhappy people—note the benefits of laughter, *"A good sense of humor can't cure all ailments, but data is mounting about the positive things laughter can do."[122]*

King Solomon had figured that out long ago. The Bible, such an amazing book, isn't it?

Laughter carries excellent short-term benefits. It helps lighten your mental load. It also induces positive physical changes in the body. Laughter can:

Stimulate many organs of the body. Laughter enhances your intake of oxygen-rich air, stimulates your heart, lungs, and muscles, and increases released endorphins in your brain. Endorphins, when released, help relieve pain, improve mood, and reduce stress.

Activates and relieves stress responders. A rollicking laugh fires up and then cools down your stress responses. It increases and decreases heart rate and blood pressure. This produces a relaxed sensation.

Soothes tension. Laughter stimulates circulation, aiding in muscle relaxation. Both help reduce some physical symptoms of stress.

Long-term Effects of Laughing

Laughter isn't just a quick pick-me-up, though. It's also good for you over the long term, producing a healthier you. Laughter may:

Improve your immune system. Negative thoughts manifest with chemical reactions, bringing stress into your system, which decreases your immune system's effectiveness. However, positive thoughts release neuropeptides that help fight stress and potentially more serious illnesses.

Relieve pain. Laughter may ease pain by causing the body to produce its own natural painkillers.

Increase personal satisfaction. Laughter can make it easier to cope with difficult situations. It also can help us connect with people.

Improve mood. Some who struggle with depression do so because of a physical illness. Laughter lessens stress, depression, anxiety, and other debilitating diseases, making us feel happier. It can also improve self-esteem.

The staff at Mayo Clinic encourages you to "find a reason to laugh."[123] Perhaps you'll need to start slowly. We don't want to overdose on laughter. Do we? Smile. That was a joke.

If you can't do a smile, begin looking for a reason to smile.

For me, suffering from FSHD Muscular Dystrophy, laughter helps ease my pain. It helps take my mind off my muscular discomfort as I focus on what's making me smile. But I have to work at it, looking for opportunities to cheer. Some days prove difficult, but if I'm able to crack a smile, it helps.

Work on Your Smilers

My grandchildren provide merry medicine. They often induce a smile in me. Anything that makes me smile, I call a 'smiler.' Search for smilers. They're out there! Just got to take time to 'smell the coffee,' as they say.

Laughter carries wonderful short-term benefits.

Some suggested smilers:

Watch children play.
View a funny movie.
Sit in a public place, observing people.
Visit an old friend.
Listen to a song from the past. I love Paul and Linda McCarthy's *Silly Love Songs*. Other examples:

Receiving kind words from someone. Smile.
A person thanking you for helping them. Smile.
Making someone else smile. Smile.
An encouraging card sent by a friend. Smile.

I save many of these, and when I'm down and troubled—as Simon and Garfunkel sang—I'll pull out one of the many cards and read them. These are God's Agape Gifts to remind me that people love and appreciate me.
Or try:

Visits to the countryside.
Watching people laugh.
Observing an older couple holding hands.
The smell of fresh brewing coffee. Did I ever mention that I LOVE COFFEE?
Spending time with loved ones.
Getting a haircut.
Receiving a gift card.
Giving a gift card.
Being around cheerful people suffering from an illness but still find goodness in life. Laughing at another's stupidity rather than making negative remarks.

A 'hello' from someone as you enter church.

Getting an alert on your phone that the thing you wanted is on sale now!

Achieving your fitness goals.

Peeking in on your sleeping children. These two words, 'sleeping children,' instantly bring back a memory of over thirty-five years ago. My three sons sleeping in the bottom bunk together with Sesame Street puppets on their hands still makes me smile.

Find those Smilers. What made you smile in the past? Rediscover it! How about a smile Wish List? Smilers that might happen in the future, like that vacation you will take. Or the anticipation of seeing friends or family. The new house you're working towards purchasing. That concert you're going to. Maybe the new car you're looking at.

I like to think about little smilers like that cappuccino I'm going to order in the morning.

Hey, makes me smile.

A movie we're going to stream tonight. The anticipation of my brother's call. He always has me laughing in stitches when we talk.

Find reasons to smile. They're out there if you just look.

Anticipate the smaller things in life that make you smile. Then, work on that smile. Go ahead. Crack the leather on your hard, sullen face and SMILE. Look for God's many evidences of goodness around you. Admiration produces a smile. There's much on the canvas of God's creation to admire.

For example, in January 1992, for the first time, concrete evidence appeared of extrasolar planets—exoplanets—orbiting a star 2300 light-years away. Today, with the Hubble and Webb Space Telescopes, we've confirmed that over 5,000 exoplanets exist, each one with its own unique characteristics.[124] This makes me smile. You do good work, God!

Sometimes, a smile comes from noticing what's going on around us. Sitting with my middle son's family over Thanksgiving, we began eating our dinner. Mashed sweet potatoes were part of the menu. It was a simultaneous moment as we all looked at the youngest family member, who'd just slopped a dollop of sweet

Search for your smilers.

potatoes on the table. As I broke out into thunderous laughter, others followed. The little mess closely resembled a plop of poop. It took quite some time for the howling to settle down.

A grin niggles a smile.

A Smile, chuckle.

A chuckle often bursts into laughter. Then, laughter becomes contagious.

When We Find It Hard to Laugh

What makes laughing so tricky for many of us? After returning from the killing fields of Kwazulu, Natal, South Africa, my soul whimpered, "What's there to laugh about?"

For those helping humanity, laughter habitually eludes them. ER nurses, firefighters, police, humanitarian workers, and missionaries—to name a few—can struggle to smile about anything. They see the worst sides of human existence. Serving as a first responder in Minnesota for eight years, first responders can find the plight of people overwhelming.

What's there to smile about, anyway?

Disturbing experiences can suck the life out of you.

A friend at the Department of Motor Vehicles, DMV, shared, "I'm so tired of rude, demanding people I find it hard to smile, ever. I hate just about everyone who walks through the door of that place."

When around a punchy, abrupt person, I try to ask myself, "Wonder what they do for a living?"

And for people who've suffered severe abuse or trauma, well… what's there to smile about, anyway? Eh?

Put Your Laughing-Feelers Out Regardless

During one of our furloughs from South Africa, we lived in Dallas, Texas, for a year. Living next to us was a young 30s-something single man. We'd see him sitting outside on his back porch from time to time.

Occasionally, I'd talk with him. He suffered from a terminal illness. He'd sit on his porch daily with a forlorn look on his drawn, thin face.

One day, I took my sons out in the backyard to practice pitching and catching. Handing out the baseball gloves, I instructed, "Ok, guys, let's be careful not to break any windows."

The backyard was a tiny little place. Our backstop was a large oak tree standing in front of the back door. After a half hour, it was Dad's turn to throw a few pitches. On my first attempt at a curve ball, the pitch went low and to the left and passed the reach of my son's glove.

That ball hit the edge of the tree trunk, ricocheted left and up into the bedroom window, shattering the glass into a dozen pieces. Our sickly neighbor broke out into a thunderous laugh as I stood with a look of disgust.

A few weeks before the young man died, he shared, "That day was the first time I've laughed in a couple of years. I really needed it. Could you break another window?" We both laughed.

Joy is Smile's Source

Unlike laughter, joy does not depend on a single event or our surroundings. It is not always dependent on how people treat us. Or our:

Station in life.
Health.
Finances.

Loneliness.

Betrayals.

Failures.

Feelings.

Or other's disappointments with us.

Joy is the realization of what is. We who enjoy a relationship with God possess a delight that overpowers this world's abundant unhappiness. It's a joy that overcomes with a calm delight, a cheerfulness, and gladness.[125]

Jesus' desire for us is that we experience full joy.

> I have told you these things so that you will be *filled with my joy.* Yes, *your joy will overflow!*
>
> Jesus — John 15:11 Emphasis Mine

Let's try to grab onto this. Jesus explained that interconnectedness with the Father provides hopeful joy. No one taught me this more than the Zulu people in South Africa.

In their plight and suffering at the height of Apartheid, my wonderful friends proved the most joyous of all. Those Christ-followers who possessed the least often appeared happier than my American friends who possessed so much. I remember thinking, "What makes these Zulu people so joyful?"

A profound, endearing joy results when we grasp the depth of God's love towards us. This joy pays dividends of happiness and contentment. This joy pays dividends of happiness and contentment.

> This High Priest of ours—*Jesus*—understands our weaknesses, for he faced all of the same testings we do, yet he did not sin.
>
> Hebrews 4:15 Italics Added

Hanging on that cross in self-powerlessness, Jesus understands what limp, lifeless arms feel like. My arms, for example. Your legs, if confined to a wheelchair like my brother Bob, who just finished his battle with FSH Muscular Dystrophy. He's free now. His body will never fail him again. He's living with Jesus.

Ever think about what heaven will be like?
Let your joy be complete.

That Jesus is your friend?
Let your joy be full.

That Jesus commands us to 'Love one another?'
Let your joy be running over.

Joy is a wonderful possession that Jesus has already secured for us.
    Let your joy be fulfilling.

And our fellowship is with the Father and with his Son, Jesus Christ. We are writing these things so that **you may fully share our joy.**

1 John 1:3b-4 Emphasis Mine

Find your joy. It's there if you can get a hold of Jesus.

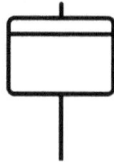

The Art of Laughter

Begin looking for smiler opportunities. Humor sits all around us if we look. Let a chuckle turn into a giggle, and a giggle into laughter. Rather than getting irritated with people, learn to smile.

Like standing in line when the person in front of me, waiting twenty minutes, just now begins the thinking process of choosing which item to order. Really? Laugh Don, laugh.

Instead of thinking, "Order stupid," just smile.

Or, instead of making my regular comment as I walk out to the car, "That's why the world needs leaders, because people are too stupid to even think ahead to order their meal." Smile, you cranky old cod.

Yeah, bet you never think like that. Right?

Or the incident at the American Airlines counter in DFW Airport while standing behind a lady who needed to rebook a canceled flight. As she ranted that her cancellation was a conspiracy of the airlines against her, I just smiled.

At the person's Starbucks, order in front of you. "Yes, I'd like a large soy milk latte, extra hot, with four shots of espresso, extra syrup, and six sugars. Oh, and a low-cal muffin, too, please." Really? Smile…

When your kids make you breakfast, leaving a wake of destruction in the kitchen. Smile, appreciate the effort.

As a little boy, a plaque hung in our kitchen with the inscription, "My kitchen is clean enough to be healthy and dirty enough to be happy." There's a smiling truth there. That plaque now hangs in our kitchen at the lake.

YouTube your favorite comedian. I love Jim Gaffigan. The guy has me in stitches most of the time. Because I'm older, comedians like Paul Lynn in the 70s, who was a world-class act, still crack me up. Others, like the Smothers Brothers from the 60s, leave me in stitches.

Read your favorite funnies. Get your favorite comic strip quote. Love Calvin and Hobbs. Or, a coffee mug with a funny saying like, "Water is coffee that hasn't reached its full potential yet."

Try smiling when getting into the shower.
What about cracking a smile when you open the fridge? Some of us will smile more than others.

Watch your favorite sitcom. For me, *Everyone Loves Raymond* was a favorite. We lived in South Africa until 2006, so they finished the series before it became available to us. Upon returning to the States, bet I've seen every episode three or four times.
I love *The Big Bang Theory*. It's a bit off-color, but I find the edginess funny. Ok, I'm not so spiritual now, right? Smile...
I grew up around edgy people until I went off to Bible College. While making new friends and having the time of my life preparing for ministry, I met some not-so-edgy stuffy people.
My Millennial sons love *The Office*. The only funny thing about the show is watching my laughing sons react to it.

Hang out with kids. Children are funny. They possess few inhibitions and are transparent.

Once, while walking into the entrance of my son's home, my grandchild approached me. I thought a big hug was coming since we hadn't seen each other in quite a while. As I readied myself for an embrace, the five-year-old stopped and asked, "Papa, are you going to die?" I replied, "Not today!" The hug followed.

That had me snickering the rest of the day.

How about making an Admiration List? I admire:

1. _____

2. _____

A Gratitude List. I'm thankful for…

1._____

2._____

Then look at your list. How about a smile?

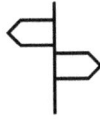

A Smiler Killer

But there's a smile killer prevalent among Christians; unforgiveness. Unforgiveness is a joy killer, and it's harmful to good mental health, too.

I've never known a happy, joyful, unforgiving person.

Forgiveness is a setting free; it's wiping a bitter soul clean. Learning to forgive encourages good mental health.

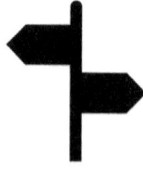

Guidepost #13

Forgive Well — Think Better

They who will not humble themselves in humbling circumstances will find their obstinacy was a nail, that will keep their misery ever fast on them without remedy.

Thomas Boston

If you **forgive** those who sin against you, your heavenly Father *will forgive you*. But if you refuse to forgive others, your Father will **not forgive** your sins.

Jesus ☐Matthew 6:14-15 Emphasis Mine

FORGIVENESS IS GOOD FOR YOUR mental health. It offers a reduction of depression, anger, stress, cardiovascular disease, and pain.

It also increases hope, compassion, and self-confidence, which helps the immune system.[126] But with many Christians struggling with mental health, I've observed a deep-seated inability to forgive.

"Forgiveness is perhaps the most challenging of all the resources available to us—and the most transformational," writes Shauna Shapiro in *Rewire Your Mind: Discover the Science + Practice of Mindfulness* (2020).

In much of my review of Positive Psychology, forgiveness is often cited as one goal for achieving optimal mental health. Hum, imagine that…. It seems I've read an ancient source that thoroughly deals with forgiveness. The Bible, it's a fantastic book, isn't it?

In the paper, *Forgiveness Can Improve Mental and Physical Health: Research Shows How to Get There, January 2017, Vol 48, No. 1,* author Kristen Weir discusses the relationship between forgiveness and mental health.

Kristen gives considerable time to the research of Everett Worthington, PhD, a professor of psychology at Virginia Commonwealth University, and his ten-year research project into forgiveness. Weir details the mental health benefits of forgiveness, asserting that the main reason for forgiveness is to release chronic stress.

Other benefits of forgiveness cited are the release of toxic anger and hostility. Whether seething anger or eruptive volcanic displays of rage, both prove hard on the physical body.

Forgiveness also increases self-esteem, helping a person change their view of themselves.

Unforgiveness takes lots of energy, and negative emotions often result as a byproduct of refusing to forgive.

If we're able to release an offense, letting it drift off the radar of our emotions, it can offer self-affirmation. Forgiveness makes us feel better about ourselves.[127]

I respect Worthington's observations because, during his ten-year study on forgiveness and its effect on mental health, a young man who never faced prosecution murdered his mother. Yet Worthington found the strength to forgive.

> 'I had applied the forgiveness model many times, but never to such a big event,' writes Worthington, 'As it turned out, I was able to forgive the young man quite quickly.'[128]

Worthington defends,

The most important part of forgiving is, once a decision to forgive is made, experiencing some positive emotions toward the person (e.g., empathy, sympathy, compassion, or love). [129]

Worthington forgave the young teenager who murdered his mother. Yet, how often do we, as Christians, refuse to forgive for much less? Worthington states forgiveness aims to "Let go of the chronic interpersonal stressors that cause us undue burden." [130]

Mayo Clinic also notes, "Forgiveness can even lead to feelings of understanding, empathy, and compassion for the one who hurt you." [131]

Wier, the paper's author citing Worthington's work on forgiveness, adds, "Outside scientific circles, many people are a bit confused about the concept."[132]

That made me chuckle. Only in the psychological community exist people who can comprehend the benefits of forgiveness. Right… so the Bible tells me so. Course, followers of Christ know that forgiveness accomplishes much more than relieving stress.

What Forgiveness Is and Is Not

Forgiveness isn't:

Forgetting what someone has done.
That there are no consequences for other's actions.
That we don't feel pain or grief.
That there's necessarily a reconciliation of relationships.
That things will always be as they once were before.[133]

Forgiveness is:

Freedom from interior bondage.
Releasing of an offense.
A setting free.

An expression of what God has done for us in Christ.[134]

Forgiveness is the discharging of another from a debt of wrongdoing, whether volitional or unintentional. It's freeing another from a payment owed or a failure to comply. A promise to not count another's sin against them.

Forgiveness is acknowledging that God will one day right all wrongs and judge those who've hurt others. How we forgive affects everything.

The Effects of Forgiveness or Lack Thereof

Forgiveness affects both our eternal standing before God and our temporal relationships with others.

It affects both the here and now and the then and there. Remember what Jesus said in Matthew chapter six?

"But if you [refuse to forgive] others, your Father *will **not forgive*** your sins."

Do you want your own wrongs forgiven? Better forgive, then.

Now, I'm not arguing against or for eternal security—once saved, always saved. Yet, I think that unforgiveness somehow affects our eternal standing with God. The nuances of this appear to be a mystery.

So, you're baptized, catechized, confirmed, and/or saved. Good for you. However, forgivelessness bears everlasting consequences, regardless.

Before you question my theology, which means you're probably a Baptist, relax. Smile. That was a joke. Well, sort of.

I'm only repeating what Jesus said. And what did Jesus say? *"If you don't forgive, you won't be forgiven."*

We can get cute and argue, "Oh, well, those words of Jesus don't apply to us today for this reason or that."

Ok, how about Paul's admonition:

Instead, be kind to each other, tenderhearted, *forgiving one another, just as God through Christ has forgiven you.*

Ephesians 4:32

Do you want forgiveness? Then, you must forgive.
No middle ground here.
Forgive, that's it.
How good of a forgiver am I?
Better than I used to be.
And honestly, still struggling with it.
How about you?
As forgiven people, we should excel in forgiving because God overlooks our sins because of Jesus.

During my pastorates in both African and American congregations, forgiveness was regularly in short supply. Some of the most egregious retributions occurred by faithful, Bible-carrying, tithing, worship-singing church members.

During my Catholic upbringing as a boy, I remember someone saying after Mass finished, "I went to confession today and did my penance, so I can still hate him when I leave church today." Friends close by laughed.

Neither is forgiveness the secular make-me-feel-good-about-myself forgiveness theology prevalent today. You know, I forgive because it's good for me. Releasing my animosities and hurt is cathartic.

That's true; partially.

But that kind of forgiveness says, "I'll release your offense so I can feel better about myself, even though I don't care about you. Forgiveness is for me. Not you. Not the both of us."

Modern psychology in studying forgiveness concludes that many benefits exist in forgiving. No argument here, but the Bible brings us to a higher place of forgiveness.

Motives for Forgiveness

The primary motive for forgiveness is obedience. We are told to do so therefore; we must.

Let's get this.

We must forgive because we're forgiven.

Christ commanded us to forgive.

The Scriptures demand that we forgive.

Living in forgiveness is the best way to model Jesus in our lives.

I forgive as I'm forgiven, and as I forgive, so am I.

"… so you must forgive others."

Colossians 3:13b

Gratitude is the flip side of forgiveness. Granting forgiveness□ absolution□to another for an injury committed is another way of saying, "Thank you, God, for forgiving me."

Remember, the *Lord forgave you*, **so you must** *forgive others.*

Colossians 3:13b Emphasis Mine

True Jesus-love requires forgiveness. We may sing, "Jesus loves me this I know…" but unless we forgive, I doubt we understand much about it.

Forgiving acknowledges that Christ overcame both our sins and others. It's often difficult to overlook another's offense. But if Christ dwells within us, the ability to forgive does, too.

> You, dear children, are from God and have overcome them, because the one who is in you is greater than the one who is in the world.
>
> I John 4:4 NIV

Forgiveness releases bitterness. I remember receiving a cup of tea from a young Zulu girl made over a paraffin stove in a mud hut in Matiwane, South Africa. The first sip sent a horrible bitter taste through my mouth. It affected my brain, too. Terrible, awful taste.

Why was it so bitter?

The soot from the burned-off paraffin made its way into the tea. Burnt paraffin ash is not tasty; I can tell you that. A smidgen of the black, grimy stuff poisons an entire cup of tea.

Unforgiveness leaves a bitter aftertaste in our souls. It turns a wholesome place into a grubby existence.

For the Bible Tells Me So

To forgive or not to forgive. Now, that is the question. What will you choose to do? Will you follow Christ's example?

> Make allowance for each other's faults, and forgive anyone who offends you. *Remember, the Lord forgave you, [so] you must forgive others.*
>
> Colossians 3:13 Emphasis and Brackets Mine

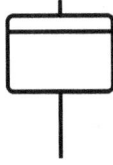

To Forgive or Not Forgive, That is the Question

My Unforgiven List

One of the boldest spiritual mental health endeavors I've ever undertaken was to make a list of those I harbored ill feelings towards. I called it *My Unforgiven List*.

I wrote down every person's name with which I had the least bit of irk. The amount of unforgiveness cluttering my soul surprised me. Then, I prioritized the lightest to the most grievous offender. For each person, I prayed a three-prong approach:

1. I thanked **God for forgiving me**.

2. I cited the person's offense.

3. I asked God to **help me forgive** that person in the same way God forgave me.

Then, I wrote after the person's name, **"I forgive you,"** and promised not to fight remembering the offense again.

Sounds good, right? Forgiving the lighter offenders wasn't difficult, but the more grievous offenses, well, that was a different story.

In my book, *To Hell, Back, and Beyond, A PTSD Journey: When Faith and Trauma Collide,* I talk much about my nemesis. At everything and anything I attempted, she opposed me. Working behind the scenes in the shadows of relationships in the church I pastored, she spread dissent about my leadership, even down to the sermons I preached on Sunday.

In my mind, I named her **Elphaba**, the Wicked Witch of the West in *The Wizard of Oz*. This is because the child actor of The Wizard of Oz grew up in the town where I pastored.

Just to think about her name tore open angry emotions. Elphaba became my greatest offender. Many souls laid waste because of her disposition. My dislike for her bordered on hatred.

It took over a year to get myself to the point of obedience to Christ and the Scriptures to forgive and mark her off *My Unforgiven List*.

When angry emotions erupted again towards her, like rewashing a dirty garment that didn't come clean in the first wash, I rinsed and repeated with forgiveness. It took many repeats of forgiveness before I could move on.

So, when compassion is a struggle, forgive. And when anger, hurt, or desire for retribution returns, rinse and repeat.

And at the core of many mentally unhealthy Christians lies unforgiveness. Apart from forgiveness, how can we ever hope to reach optimal mental health?

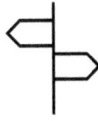

Much of what we're talking about centers upon how we think about ourselves, others, and what's going on around us. How we interpret events and act upon them.

Thinking influences behavior.
Behavior shows how we think.
How we think becomes the actual fight.
We win or lose in our minds.
The battle is between our ears.

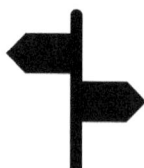

Guidepost #14

The Real Battle Happens Between Our Ears

Many people go looking for wool and come back shorn.

— Don Quixote

IN THE 17TH CENTURY, Miguel de Cervantes, regarded as the most excellent writer in Spanish literature, wrote *The Ingenious Gentleman Don Quixote of La Mancha.*

Cervantes' masterpiece is one of the most translated books in the world. The story concerns a noble Hidalgo who loses his mind reading chivalric romances. Deciding to become a knight, he enlists a subsistence farmer to become his squire.[135]

The main character, Don Quixote, and his peasant squire enter the 'dangerous countryside,' tilting and charging at imaginary foes.

On the battlefield, Quixote sees evil giants, which are nothing more than a group of windmills. Charging at full gallop, he impales a windmill's sail, knocking himself and the horse to the ground. In Quixote's imaginary in-between-the-ears battle, he suffers actual physical injuries.[136]

So, too, imaginary battles simmering in our minds often injure us. Invented encounters we thrash about in our heads wound us and others. Then, there's the spiritual carnage that follows in our souls.

Sometimes, our imaginary battles begin as intrusive thoughts urging us into a hostile act towards someone, something, or ourselves. Perhaps it surprises you that the Apostle Paul spoke of dealing with intrusive thoughts?

> Casting down arguments and every high thing that exalts itself against the knowledge of God, *bringing every thought* into *captivity to the obedience of Christ…*
>
> 2 Corinthians 10:5 NKJV Emphasis Mine

The biggest battle you'll ever fight is between your ears. There, the windmills of fear, anger, abuse, apprehension, doubts, mistrust, or addictions prepare for battle. What is your windmill?

Fill in the blank: My windmill is _____.

When was the last time you charged an inaccurate perception, issue, or person who either wasn't real or lacked accuracy? Deluded windmills we nurture in our minds that spin deficits in our thinking. Well, those windmills affect our mental health.

Battle of the Mind

Where do such windmills originate? Sometimes, our windmills come from negative remarks.

An abandonment.
Betrayal.
A possible upcoming encounter.

The biggest battle you'll ever fight is within your mind.

An experience.

A hurt.

What we believe someone said about us. Such windmills lay waste to our lives in inaccurate arenas within the mind.

Let's look again at Paul's words:

We *demolish* arguments and every pretension that sets itself up against the knowledge of God, and we *take captive* every thought to make it obedient to Christ.

2 Corinthians 10:5 NIV Emphasis Mine

Demolish.

Taking a captive.

Warlike talk.

Capturing mental imaging that is not accurate or an outright lie. We struggle within ourselves as we fight foes that exist only in the mind.

When's the last time you pined away, lost in thought processes of a past event, or perceived confrontation of the future? Worrying about something that never happened? Maybe confronting someone you thought spoke ill of you, finding out the opposite was true? Or a conflict made bigger than it actually was. We lean towards this often, don't we?

Part of CBT—Cognitive Behavior Therapy—is to help people think differently, eliminating those spinning blades of imaginary battles in the mind. The Bible nailed this down centuries ago:

Don't copy the behavior and customs of this world, but let God **transform** you into a new person by **changing the way you think**.

Romans 12:2a

My application of this verse is to vanquish windmills through accurate thinking. Inaccurate thoughts often become idols of our hearts. Imps of the mind that, like in the Lord of the Rings, run amuck in our imaginary caves of Mordor.

Often, while listening to someone rehearse their thoughts about an incident, I'll gently inquire, "How accurate is what you just said?" After their response, sometimes I'll add, "How much of that is your own windmill, and how much of it is accurate truth?"

Often, we base our thinking upon falsehoods, presuppositions, or suspicions that don't reflect reality. Lies from the Father of Lies. Fabrications like:

No one really cares about me.
That person is out to get me.
Everything is against me.
All men are predators.
All women are deceitful.
I can't trust anyone anymore.
I never get a break.
What's that person saying about me?
Life really sucks.
Why is everyone out to get me?
I can't get ahead no matter what I do.
When I see that person again, I'm going to…
Why do they get all the breaks?
Nothing lucky ever comes my way.

Get rid of your windmills. Their idols of the heart.

Doesn't matter what I do.

That church.

That which

Those imaginary battles simmering in your head can cause real damage.

Those missionaries.

My missions agency.

Those team members.

That pastor.

My Ex.

Those 'friends.'

Cranial foes put into motion, spinning blades of unjustifiable anger, resentment, and bitterness. Rage churns within as we war against that which inaccurately reflects reality.

A beginning irritation that turns frustration into fury.

A perceived hostility that doesn't exist.

A brewing animosity over spoken words, judging a person's intention, turning them from a noncombatant into a foe. *Psychology Today* offers some help here. Consider:

Cognitive Distancing. You notice people looking up at you in a restaurant. Rather than thinking, "Why are they looking at me?" think, "They seem to enjoy a pleasant discussion.

Replace irrational thoughts with rational thinking. Instead of, "I bet I'm going to lose my job," substitute with, "Let's see what's going to happen, and then I'll adjust."

Again, this isn't new to the Bible. Paul instructed,

…**put off your old self**, which belongs to your former manner of life and is corrupt through deceitful desires, and to be renewed in the spirit of your minds, and to **put on the new self**, created after the likeness of God in true righteousness and holiness. Ephesians 4:22-24 ESV Emphasis Mine

Use a Mantra. A pastor friend encourages his members to repeat, "God is good. All the time, God is good."

Or, let's say you're sitting in traffic on the freeway during a hot day. Instead of, "Why doesn't that idiot in front of me get going?" Think, "It's good to have air-conditioning today."

When fearful or negative, Say, "Life is good." Or, "It's is OK."

Practice repeating such phrases when your mind conjures up mental windmill's cutting blades.

Focus on the Present. What's happened, happened. There is nothing you can do to change it. What will happen, will happen. We can't predict the future.

Focus on the present. What's happening now. This kicks your prefrontal neocortex—the brain's rational part—into control over your sometimes inaccurate, overreactive limbic system.

It doesn't mean you're blindly unaware of what is happening, happened, or might occur in the future, but focusing on the present helps you deal with now-situations rationally.

Write Things Down. Writing engages the brain's rational part, taking the mind off what's troubling you. Once your thoughts are calm, reconsider your thinking.

Breathe. 'Breathing shifts your fight-or-flight response to a relaxed response of the parasympathetic nervous system.'[137]

Count to five. Breathe deeply through your nose, hold your breath for five seconds, then slowly release the air through your mouth with pursed lips. This helps relax the body by taking in oxygen-rich air. It settles the mind as thoughts concentrate on breathing.[138]

It takes practice to control your thoughts. Work at it. Replace those Windmills of Worse Case Scenarios with truth-thoughts.

Scripture often talks about refocusing our thinking upon God. This helps control our fears, worries, and anger, and quiets the soul, looking away from our anxieties.

You will *keep in perfect peace* all who **trust in you**,
all whose **thoughts are fixed** on you!

Isaiah 26:3 Emphasis Mine

'Trust,' be confident in someone or something; here, the Creator. 'Fixed,' literally to take hold of, lean against, or rest upon,[139] causing the orbital prefrontal cortex to focus upon a fixed point—God. 'Perfect peace,' literally shalom shalom, watches over us.

Focusing upon prayer rather than windmills of doubt:

Don't worry <u>about anything</u>; ***instead,*** <u>pray about everything</u>.
[Tell God] *what you need*, and [thank him] for all he has done.

Then you will experience God's peace, which exceeds anything we can understand. His *<u>peace will **guard** your hearts and minds</u>* as you live in Christ Jesus.

Philippians 4:6-7 Emphasis Mine

Verse twenty-four here is power-packed. The word 'guard' comes from a military word in Paul's language. It carries the idea of garrisoning, fortifying, or barricading to protect. God's peace can garrison our hearts and minds with inexplicable peace rather than foundering in unhealthy thoughts and angst.

175

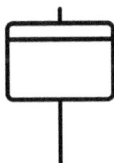

What About Your Windmills?

Consider the windmills you're currently chasing. You know, those anxiety-producing thoughts lurking about in your soul. Describe them on paper or in a journal.

Examine your thinking. How many of your mental inclinations are healthy? What thoughts are based upon unsubstantiated suspicions, self-focused windmills, slaying your mind and soul?

Keep a journal of your thoughts. Be honest. Describe your emotions about an event or person. Be precise. Ask yourself:

How accurate are my thoughts?
How well do I know that person?
What conclusions do my thoughts bring me to?
Do I possess complete knowledge of that person or event?
What is the effect of these feelings on my mind and body?
How do my windmills affect my sleep?
How do they affect others?
Are my thoughts healthy or detrimental?
Do they encourage or damage relationships?

Do they make friends or enemies?

What thinking do I need to change?

Who do I need to seek help with my mental processing?

Seek forgiveness from?

Grant forgiveness, too?

And the biggie:

Where is Christ in Your Thinking?

Spend a month recording your thoughts for the day. No matter how trivial, write them down. Then, place those thoughts before you. Look at your journal, smartphone, laptop, or wherever you've recorded your thoughts. Then, have a little talk with Jesus:

Jesus, you've already paid to remove my windmills. But I struggle to let go.

Once again, I place all my anger, anxieties, and worries before you, asking that you free my mind and soul from these thoughts that cause me so much angst.

I forgive _____ (Name the Person) for what he/she/they/ did to me.

Free me from my fear of _____ .

Take away my anger of/with/about _____ .

Unchain me from my constant worry of _____ .

Rid me of my constant battle with unhealthy thoughts. Name those thoughts. Amen.

As your windmills reappear, rinse and repeat as needed.

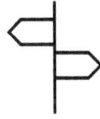

Physical health can also take a heavy toll on mental health. This is an area we often ignore.

Our primary passions push physical needs to the back of our busy schedules. We sacrifice sound physical health practices for something we deem more important, bringing unhealthy repercussions upon ourselves.

We go down with the ship that we've unknowingly scuttled ourselves. When we ignore our health, inevitably, mental health declines.

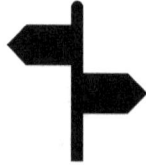

Guidepost #15

Healthy Body—Healthier Mind

SERVING OTHERS CAN TAKE A HEAVY toll on both mental and physical health. This seems especially true with pastors, missionaries, caregivers, or those involved in EMS, policing, nursing, and firefighting.

For missionaries, there's no avoiding the diseases of the Third World. When entering a new country for service, bodies unfamiliar with the new environment often fall ill.

I remember my trips to India from South Africa. Landing in Mumbai, unfamiliar smells immediately assaulted my senses. Natural everyday surroundings so familiar to local people brought me unpleasantries and illness with frustrating rapidity.

When my guide instructed, "Don't eat that or don't drink this."

I responded, "But you're drinking that beverage and eating the food."

With a chuckle came the reply, "Yes, but we're Indian. You're not from here. Trust me, I've watched many pastors and missionaries come to India who refused to follow my advice. They get sick. Some end up in hospital." Then, smirking, he added, "You don't want to spend time in an Indian hospital, do you?"

One morning, out in the middle of Kolhapur, a Nescafe Coffee shop stood on the corner. Now, I recognized that from South Africa; Nescafe Coffee. Soon, it was discovered that the similarity between the two coffees existed only in the name.

Entering with a young apprentice guide, I ordered my coffee with cream and sugar. By evening, sickness ruled my body. It didn't bother the young guide who sat with me drinking the same beverage, but I thought death was imminent.

The following day, as we all gathered—teachers, students, and workers—an announcement came from the leader. "Dr. Mingo may not drink or eat anything other than what we put in front of him."

Bang! Well deserved. After a week, I was better, and my teaching continued.

Here's the thing. No matter your diligence, you're probably going to fall ill. Most cross-cultural workers who spend considerable time in the field learn to live with diseases that disproportionately affect developing countries.

With clergy, constant stress, caring for others' souls, administration of the church, exposure to congregants' complaints, and attacks by spiritual saboteurs take their toll on the body. Over the long haul, physical health declines.

As a missionary, visiting hundreds of churches throughout the United States and trying to raise our support over the years, I often wondered, "What's wrong with so many of these pastors?"

Upon accepting the position as Lead Pastor in Minnesota, it began to make unfortunate sense. The pressure crushed me. Unprepared for the challenges of managing an inherited dysfunctional staff with inept deacon and elder boards, it felt like a never-ending episode of *The Walking Dead.*

We regularly fail to care for their physical health. Overweight, sleep deprived, and stressed with endless activity leave many constantly depleted. Often, preventable illnesses arise from the lack of solid self-care. And here's a fact:

People with chronic illness are far more likely to struggle with their mental health. Some risk factors in mental health are directly attributable to physical health.[140]

Nearly one in three people with a long-term physical health condition also have a mental health problem, most often depression or anxiety. [141]

Research shows that people with mental health issues are more likely to suffer from preventable physical health conditions such as heart disease.[142]

Anxiety or Physical Dysfunction

For me, what I thought for years was anxiety proved partly a health issue. Unbeknownst to me, my weakening arms were not from the aging process. When, during a Christmas get-together with family, I reached for a pitcher of water, failing to lift it from the table, I knew it was time to seek medical attention.

After six months of testing and genetic blood work, the diagnosis came back: Facioscapulohumeral Muscular Dystrophy (FSHD). And it didn't stop there. After an MRI of my heart, we discovered that my heart was also affected.

Don't you realize that your body is the temple of the Holy Spirit... You do not belong to yourself... you must honor God with your body.

1 Corinthians 6:19a-20b

Upon beginning a regimen of medication for my heart, guess what? Reduced anxiety. The best thing you can do for yourself is get a complete physical yearly.

Take care of your body, which is the temple, dwelling place, of the Holy Spirit.

That Forest Lake Pastor

Once, Kathy and I stopped in Forest Lake, Minnesota, at Perkins for breakfast. As we ate, two paramedics entered, making their way to the back of the Restaurant. There, they attended to a pastor who collapsed and lay on the floor semi-conscious.

As they placed the ill pastor onto a gurney, he objected, "Do I have to go to the hospital? I'm a pastor and don't have insurance."

By law, you can't force treatment upon an objecting patient. With that, the paramedics left. Twenty minutes later, that Forest Lake pastor cautiously made his way towards the door.

That following Sunday, he stood before a congregation that didn't care enough to provide their pastor and his family health insurance. Something every member of his leadership team enjoyed.

Know When to Fold 'Em or Hold 'Em

The late western singing legend Kenny Rogers sang a hit song, *The Gambler*. The song's chorus, referring to playing a hand of poker, went:

You've got to know when to hold 'em
Know when to fold 'em
Know when to walk away
And know when to run…

We must play the hand we're dealt, but let's not be stubborn or foolish. Sometimes, stubbornness is not our friend. *Don't ignore your physical health.* Know when to hold your position and when to seek help.

A few years ago, Kathy and I met a young Vietnamese missionary. She shared her ministry and impressed us in many ways. Later, we heard from a close friend that she had found a lump in her breast. However, she was far too busy to seek medical help, and as a newly arrived immigrant to the United States, her medical options were also limited.

Counsel came from poor-thinking friends who told her that her faith, if strong enough, would heal her. At thirty-five years old, she died. That small lump metastasized, taking her life.

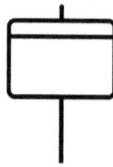

Time for a Checkup

How's your:

- Get enough sleep?
- Find the time to exercise?
- Pay attention to what you eat and drink?
- Take some mind-rest time for yourself?
- Accept help when it's offered?
- Plan something you look forward to?
- Learn relaxation techniques?
- Find something you like to do. And then do it?

How well do you care for your mind?

- What do you put into your brain?
- What about your internet, TV, and social media habits?
- Unhealthy conversations?
- Who can you talk with about your struggles?

What's your soul care like?

-   How do you practice generosity?
-   What anger do you harbor?
-   When do you spend time in nature?
-   What fears control you?
-   What about journaling?
-   How are your spiritual disciplines?
-   How often do you go to God and talk about the needs of your soul?
-   Who do you need to seek, asking for their forgiveness?
-   Who might you need to grant forgiveness to?

People with chronic illnesses are far more likely to struggle with their mental health.

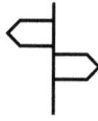

In all this self-care talk, an unhealthy preoccupation with ourselves may creep upon us. That's when we focus so much on our mental health that we never get past our struggles, becoming primarily about ourselves.

The call to every Christ-follower is to live above a self-absorbed. To take up our cross daily and follow Christ.

> *Then he said to the crowd, "If any of you wants to be my follower, you must give up your own way, take up your cross daily, and follow me.*
>
> Luke 9:23

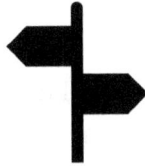

Guidepost #16

Live Above a Self-Absorbed Life

A trait I've noticed among those struggling with their mental health is an incessant preoccupation with self.

SOMETIMES IN TRYING TO CARE for our mental health, an unintentional self-fixation develops.

Panic attacks or depression are not uncommon among missionaries giving their all in serving others. I'd rather burn out than rust out is the mantra. And burnout, they do.

I thought, "What's the difference? Either way, you're out."

Pastors stand front and center. They're the leaders, shepherds. People look to them for guidance and spiritual sustenance. They become continual fixers of other's problems. People come expecting the pastor to walk on water on their behalf. Constantly entering the emotional waters of other's difficulties, clergy drown in their own mental frailty.

Sitting within the church, numerous attendees struggle with secret mental health problems. Often, members of my church came to me with complex issues. Complications that sucked every smidgin of energy out of their lives.

Their dilemmas proved difficult for me to leave at the office. At home, my thoughts kept circling around other's problems.

A family whose son's irrational self-destructing behavior required them to admit him into a psychiatric ward at the hospital.

The burial of a son, accidentally shot in the woods by a brother during hunting.

Adult children move an aged parent suffering from Alzheimer's into their ill-equipped house.

A single mom working three jobs and still not earning enough to care for her family.

When such events push us to the end of our coping capabilities, self-focus becomes necessary initially, asking, "What's wrong with me?

Mental health concerns require a close look to assess the cause of a person's mental health condition.

This is cause-and-effect.

What Causes My…

Take a person battling with high levels of anxiety. What becomes their initial focus?

Why am I so anxious?
How can I ease what's causing my anxiousness?
What do I need to do to deal with this condition?

Initially, scrutinizing the problem is essential. However, it's not a healthy place to remain. It's a beginning, not an end. Eventually, we need to look beyond ourselves, our injuries, trauma, and problems lest we become our own chief preoccupation.

At least, that's the way it worked for me. As long as I focused solely on my PTSD, it became more intrusive and destructive. Eventually, I learned to look towards managing my PTSD rather than obsessing over it.

How many conversations I've had with missionaries, pastors, and church members who can't move beyond:

Here's what happened to me.
This is what he/she/ they did to me.
You know what it feels like to…?
Do you know how that makes me feel?
Let me tell you about my…
I'm this or that way because of…
I just can't stop thinking about…
I can't get past it...
The memories keep coming back…

Hyper-fixation and self-preoccupation develop. *We become constant problem-thinkers rather than problem-solvers.*

Rehearsing a perceived betrayal, for example, prevents us from releasing an offense.

Recovery becomes impossible because of an obsession with 'what happened to me, what I'm feeling, or my condition.'

A fault finding, to the minutest degree that overcompensates for our own deficits, constantly pointing out the imperfections in others.

The divorce you can't let go of.

Resentment for a physical handicap you must live with for the rest of your life.

A career advancement that you deserved but went to another.

Living in an unfair world that treats you unfairly.

Over-inflating your worth, or under-inflating your value.

> *...I focus on this one thing: Forgetting the past and looking forward to what lies ahead...*
>
> Philippians 13b

Self-Obsessions

A young missionary couple returning from an extended internship on the field sat before me. Anxieties weighed upon them. With a list of grievances against an older missionary couple that hosted them, they went into verbal tirades.

A young missionary couple returning from an extended internship on the field sat before me. Anxieties weighed upon them. They went into verbal tirades with a list of grievances against an older missionary couple that hosted them.

It's a question I often ask missionaries struggling to get along with other missionaries, "What does this missionary you're struggling with do well?"

The young missionary trainees sitting before me answered, "Nothing."

I responded, "Nothing? There isn't one thing they did well?"

"Nope. Absolutely not," came the reply.

My questions zeroed in on the young couples' lack of gratitude, overcritical attitude, and self-absorbing mindsets. "How long have they served on the field?" I asked.

One launched, "WELL! That's all they've done is live there!"

"For how long?" I asked.

"Well, thirty-five years, I guess," came the reply.

Leaning back, I reflected, "Isn't one of the biggest challenges of a cross-cultural worker to make the place you serve in your home?"

For another hour, I did my best to help the young couple see their problem which was, in fact, not with the older missionary couple who hosted them but within themselves.

Even when serving others we can become mostly about ourselves.

Their self-adulation, critical, over-inflated attitude put the spotlight upon only themselves. Their way seemed righteous, and everyone else was inept. They resigned from missionary service shortly afterward, citing everyone else as the reason for leaving their calling.

This scene plays out repeatedly. Missionaries who, upon the moment they land on the tarmac in the country they intend to serve, see only the shortcomings of everyone else but themselves.

Pastors, enduring the worst in a few of their congregants, quit their callings with wounded spirits, believing the entire church opposed them. Unmet expectations of others towards us can hurt, and then we think we're unable to move past them.

In all this lay the seeds of a self-centered mindset. Even when serving others, we can become mostly about ourselves. What we want. How others must react. How I must be treated. Why they must follow me. An overly critical spirit, inspiring self-absorption, taints our actions and attitudes. Add to all this, a bona fide mental illness and thinking can become toxic.

Preoccupations' Necessities and Dangers

Excessive self-focused attention is considered by many experts to be the *core of a number of anxiety disorders* such as panic disorder, OCD, social and sexual anxiety. [143]

Many grappling with their mental health simply don't know how to overcome an injury, incident, or malady of life and move past it.

Why did he/she/they do that to me?
When will I ever be able to be around people again?
What if they found out about my condition?
What makes it hurt so much?
How come I'm angry all the time?
Why am I sad all the time?
What's happening to me?
Why can't I sleep?
How can I ever be happy again?
Why did they hurt me?
How come God doesn't answer my prayers?
Why did my child die?
What made my spouse leave me?
How come I'm sick all the time?
Why don't people like me?
I'll never overcome this addiction?
How can I ever trust anyone again?

> *Eventually, we need to look beyond ourselves lest we become our own chief occupation.*

For those who criticize a problem-centric approach, I argue, "How can you help a person deal with an issue if both counselor and counselee don't understand the problem?"

You can offer Bible verses for anxiety, but what's causing the anxiety? Finding the source of a person's anxiety and then targeting it with Scripture, I've seen, is far more effective.

I'm anxious about _____. Ok, let's look at what Scripture says about that, shall we?

Yes, Jesus is that answer, but Christ's approach to people often began with questions. In fact, Jesus asked hundreds of questions, which were recorded in the Gospels. Yet, he answered very few of them.[144]

Excessive Self-Absorption

Obsessing causes adverse effects:

> ... many other personality disturbances can be seen as involving self-absorption (histrionic, paranoid, avoidant, dependent, and obsessive-compulsive).... feeling threatened, vulnerable, and insecure—which gets at the heart of why self-absorption is such a common characteristic in those who harbor profound doubts about themselves that it impairs their everyday functioning. [145]

The challenge becomes differentiating narcissism—people overly focused on themselves—from those suffering from mental impairment, physical ailments, or both. Even with bona fide mental health issues, often the biggest challenge is to not constantly focus on a mental disorder.

Years ago, in North Minneapolis, during the hot summer months, my youngest brother Bob would ride around the streets of his disadvantaged neighborhood in his motorized wheelchair, handing out cold bottles of water to those in need. He called it his ministry.

When a tornado hit North Minneapolis, Minnesota, where he lived, he wheeled around the devastated neighborhood, giving out those cold water bottles to anyone in need. Months earlier, he had solicited dozens of cases of water from individuals, friends, churches, and businesses. All this while confined to a wheelchair.

Bob often told me, "This wheelchair doesn't confine me but helps love and serve others."

For his outstanding contributions to the tornado relief effort, he received the Minnesota State Council on Disability's Emergency Preparedness Award in 2009.

He rarely complained. Often, he joked and laughed. All this while confined to a wheelchair in immense pain.

After learning of my diagnosis, he encouraged me, "The way you get through this Don is that when you wake up, find something in which to be thankful. Then, focus upon that the rest of the day."

In hospice, some of his last words to me were, "Now, after I'm gone, remember to look at the low-hanging fruit of gratitude. It's up to you to pick it from the tree or let it fall to the ground of ingratitude. If you carry the fruit of gratitude daily, you'll focus on God's goodness and the friends he's surrounded you with rather than just your pain and yourself."

Within a few days, Bob departed his wretched physical being, gaining a faultless body that would never again fail him.

There comes a point when we must learn to look beyond our woes. That's not to say ignore them. Take care of yourself. Do the best you can. Deal with your issues. But also learn to look beyond them lest your life exists only in the hardships and troubles of life.

And just how do we do that?

Self Is Not the Primary Focus of a Christ-Centered Life

Yes, the second greatest commandment is to 'Love your neighbor as yourself.' However, I don't think Jesus was saying to make self the center of our affections. More like, "Treat others the same way you'd like them to treat you."

Jesus spoke about our tendency to concern ourselves primarily with ourselves.

Then he said to the crowd, 'If any of you wants to be my follower, you must give up your own way, take up your cross daily, and follow me.'

Jesus — Luke 9:27

Philippians 2:3-4 gives good instruction here:

Don't be selfish; Don't try to impress others. Don't look out only for your own interests, Take an interest in others, too. Be humble, thinking of others as better than yourself.

What About You?

With mental health challenges, we initially ask, "What is happening?" Within ourselves, we sense a problem. While necessary in determining the root of a cause, self must not remain in a fetal position wrapped around its tragedies and suffering. We need to move forward, managing meaningful lives rather than cocooning ourselves in our hurts, struggles, and disabilities.

Our struggles are not random misfortunes but buoys marking direction in the waves of life's turbulence.

That's the learning curve I've experienced with my Muscular Dystrophy and PTSD. "What's the problem?" was necessary. That was a beginning; not the end.

It's not where I'm going to stay. It only gives an entry point to understand and learn how to cope with my ailments, not surrender to them.

Learn to live beyond yourself. Some of the most amazing people I've known are those who reach out to others while in intense anguish.

An alcoholic encourages another struggling with drinking to live a life of abstinence.

A single mom whose husband abandoned her encourages another single mom to survive without her ex-husband. Actually, overheard that conversation between two women the other day in a Kroger's Grocery Store.

194

See your stigma, struggle, illness, or disability as an opportunity. Michael J. Fox, the famous *Back to the Future* actor, now stricken with Parkinson's Disease, shares, "Gratitude makes optimism sustainable."[146]

Your situation affords you opportunities that 'healthy people' rarely get; appreciation for living and helping other strugglers like you.

Focus on healthy living. Learn not to obsess. Refuse to live in an ocean of self-loathing, self-pity, and self-obsession.

> He comforts us in all our troubles so that we can comfort others. When they are troubled, we will be able **to give them the same comfort** God has given us.
>
> 2 Corinthians 1:4 Emphasis Mine

Boast about – sure, I'll talk about my issue! How to overcome. Where it helps more than it hurts. How it teaches an appreciation for life. The reason is that I'm the lucky one who's learning to live with more purpose.

Take pleasure in – yep! I'll take pleasure in my pain. Well, try anyway. Pain can lend itself to a perspective otherwise unattainable.

So, the power of Christ can work through me. I know it's difficult to see, but at our weakest point, we can identify with Christ. Paul said that Christ became the strongest person in his life at his weakest point. 1 Corinthians 12:9-10

Comfort – as we learn to be comforted, we can comfort others. Here, right here, in this verse, lies the purpose for our pain.

How can you help others struggling like yourself?

What makes you an overcomer?

Where is Christ in your suffering?

195

Purpose. That's the key. Seeing that our struggles are not random misfortunes but buoys marking a purposeful direction in life's waves of turbulence.

If you're a Jesus-follower, understand there are no accidents. God didn't just wake up one day and say, "Oh, sorry, missed that one! My bad."

There's a purpose in pain. In purpose comes meaning, and in meaning, fulfillment lies within our grasp. Purpose brings mental prosperity. Knowing what to do with your 'thorn in the flesh' uses your pain for gain. Purpose transforms misery into ministry. It turns suffering into service.

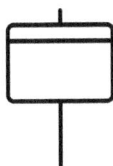

The Good Thing About Weakness

It's in weakness we can discover ourselves in a new way. 2 Corinthians 12:9-10

Like Elijah, God can meet you in your cave of despair. Then, you can leave that damp, dark place with renewed purpose. I Kings 19:9-18

Your weakness:

How can your weakness become your new strength? Where can you see Christ in your mental health struggles?

How about listing some **possible new strengths?**

1.

2.

3.

> *Knowing what to do with your 'thorn' in the flesh turns pain into purpose.*

Remember:

This High Priest (Jesus) of ours **<u>understands our weaknesses</u>**, for he faced all of the same testings we do, yet he did not sin.

Hebrews 4:15 Brackets and Emphasis Mine

Jesus understands. Go to him often in your pain. He's felt the same pain you're experiencing, right now.

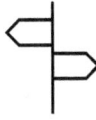

Choose the Way You Want to Live

Ultimately, the attitude you choose determines how you live.

See yourself as a victim. You become a victim.

See yourself as helpless. You become helpless.

See yourself as unlucky. Guess what? You're unlucky.

A victim of circumstances? Then circumstances dictate your life.

Life's unfair? Yep, but living in a life's-unfair-to-me mindset sours disposition toward self and others. 'Why me' leads you only back to yourself.

Will you choose to become a Victor or a Victim?

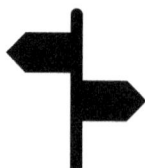

Guidepost #17

Become a Victor

SITTING WITH A GROUP OF MILITARY VETERANS, two kinds of people stood out. The first group lamented their plight. Struggling with substance abuse, they 'owed' to PTSD; many had lost their marriages.

Others struggled to hold down jobs. Some living on well-deserved disability benefits suffered from mental and physical deficits. A few experienced living homeless on the streets.

Most in the first group sat with grimaces on their faces, dripping with hopelessness and anger. They were victims. Mental casualties of the harsh realities of war, attributing their misfortunes to military life. Sullied attitudes of loss and misfortune filled the room.

Now, a few with similar war experiences distinguished themselves. All suffered from PTSD—sleepless nights, night terrors, hyper noise sensitivity, anger—and all the rest that comes with it.

But with them, overcoming marked divergence in their thinking and actions.

These men strove to overcome their deficits and mental maladies, determined to move forward. They chose to be victors rather than victims.

It's Not Fair

What happened to you, what happened to me, and what happens to others appears to occur unequally. That's not fair.

It's a crummy reality of life.

But regardless of injury, illness, health, or mental ailment, you will make a choice to either move forward or wallow in victimhood, self-pity, and despair.

Generalizing life with continual feelings of victimhood affects our relationships and quality of life. Our identity reduces to that of the victim.[147] Victim-thinking projects, "I am a person of misfortune. Unlucky in life. Mistreated. "

It's natural to acknowledge hurt; this or that happened to me. Healthy, perhaps, initially, in understanding the ramifications of what happened. Processing, while painful, is necessary for good mental health.

But there comes a fork in our mental roads. *One is that of an overcomer, the other leads towards becoming a casualty.*

As a casualty, victimhood becomes our identity. Who we project to others. The worst things in life.

"Hi, I'm _____, and this happened to me."

I'm learning this with both my PTSD and FSHD Muscular Dystrophy. When I continually talk about my pain, disadvantage, and all the facets of suffering, people know me not as Don but as 'the guy with PSTD and MD.' Most mistake it for MS, but that's another issue altogether.

It becomes a self-destructive way to live. I become known as a victim because I act like a victim. And here's another discovery: people tend not to want to be around that kind of person.

They don't like or cannot hear of others' pain. That's why many struggling with their mental health enjoy few friends. *American Scientific* notes that researchers found those with a victimhood mindset displayed four main behaviors:

(1) constantly seeking recognition for one's victimhood,
(2) moral elitism,
(3) lack of empathy for the pain and suffering of others, and
(4) frequently ruminating about past victimization. [148]

What choice will you make?

Better Questions than 'Why Me?'

How can I move forward?
Who do I need to seek for help?
What resources might be helpful?
When does that program begin?
What will it take to succeed?
What professional help do I need?
Which church can I involve myself with that might help me?
Where is that recovery group located?
How can I see God's presence in all of this?
Where does the Bible speak to my issues?
How might prayer help?

And for me, the biggie is, "How can I use my deficits for the benefit of others and myself?"

In finding purpose in pain, meaning in misery, tranquility in trauma, and gratitude in grievance, life wraps itself in significance, appreciation, and worth.

In Christ, We Are Victors

Even in the tough stuff of life, we can become more than survivors:

No, in all these things *we are more than conquerors* through him who loved us. For I am convinced that neither death nor life, neither angels nor demons, neither the present nor the future, nor any powers, neither height nor depth, nor anything else in all creation, will be able to separate us from the love of God that is in Christ Jesus our Lord.

Romans 8:37-39 NIV Emphasis Mine

Become a Survivor rather than Victim

Yes, you probably were a victim, but don't be one now. It's really a choice. Isn't it? Maybe a grueling process, but still a choice. And it's a decision only you can make. Once you make that choice, it becomes yours. You own it, and no one can take it away from you. You decide, "NO MORE!"

Will you live as a victim, or will you gain mastery over your condition, managing yourself to a better you? Become an overcomer. Become a better you. And remember:

You, dear children, are from God and **have overcome** them, because the *one who is in you is greater than the one who is in the world.*

Other Books by Don Mingo

Son Risings – *Discovering and Caring for the Real You.*

So, You Want to Be A Missionary: *Essential Considerations.*

The Cross-Cultural Worker's Spiritual Survival Guide: *14 Survival Tips to Help You Thrive in Your Calling.*

To Hell, Back and Beyond: A PTSD Journey – *When Faith and Trauma Collide.*

The Faith Principle – *4 Secrets to Making Your Faith Work Again.*

Slaying the Dragon Within: *5 Steps to Help Christians GetOut of Porn* – *A Discipleship Approach*

Slaying the Dragon Within Workbook in Color: *5 Steps to Help Christians Get Out of Porn* – *A Discipleship Approach*

Slaying the Dragon Within Workbook in B & W: *5 Steps to Help Christians Get Out of Porn* – *A Discipleship Approach*

Just Get Me Through This Day! *Balancing Career, family, relationships, and the IMPORTANT STUFF OF LIFE*

Get Your Life Back! Journal. *A 21-week addiction renewal journal.*

Author's Biography

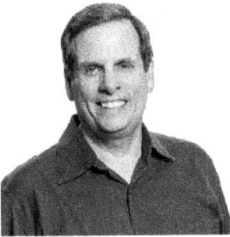

Don served with his wife Kathy for twenty-two years as missionaries in South Africa. He then pastored two churches in Minnesota. Currently, Don and Kathy serve in Member Care to missionaries and pastors around the world.

Don holds a bachelor's degree from Baptist Bible College in Springfield, Missouri, a Master of Theology Degree from Bethany Theological Seminary in Dothan, Alabama, and a Master and Doctor of Ministry Degree from Luther Rice Seminary in Lithonia, Georgia.

He also holds several certifications and training in Critical Incident Stress Management, Chaplaincy, Life Coaching, Depression Recovery, and other disciplines.

Don and Kathy are professional life coaches who have received training from the Professional Christian Coaching Institute.

Don is the CEO of Mingo Coaching Group. He and his wife, Kathy, head Missionary to Missionary Care, which offers coaching, care, and counsel to missionaries, pastors, and leaders worldwide.

Don has severe PTSD and Facioscapulohumeral Muscular Dystrophy. This uniquely enables him and Kathy, his wife and care provider, to encourage others.

---

[1] Jackson, Dory. "Michael J. Fox Says 'Gratitude Makes Optimism Sustainable' While Living with Parkinson's Disease." Peoplemag. PEOPLE, November 30, 2021https://people.com/tv/michael-j-fox-gratitude-makes-optimism-sustainable-parkinsons-disease/

[2] Hartz, S. (n.d.). The Truth About Missionaries and Depression. Sarita Hartz. Retrieved October 3, 2022, from http://www.saritahartz.com/tags/coaching/

[3] (U.S.), O. M. F. I. (2021, December 15). *5 questions not to ask missionaries with mental health struggles.* OMF (U.S.). Retrieved April 18, 2023, from https://omf.org/us/how-to-care-for-missionaries-with-mental-health-struggles/

[4] Rance, Valerie. (2014). Trauma and the Mental Health of the Missionary: Effects, Coping and Missionary Care. Encounter: Journal for Pentecostal Ministry. 11.1-16.

[5] Encounter: Journal for Pentecostal Ministry, Summer 2014, Vol. 11 Trauma and the Mental Health of the Missionary: Effects, Coping and Missionary Care Valerie Rance, Ph.D. in Intercultural Studies student Assemblies of God Theological Seminary

[6] Mayo Foundation for Medical Education and Research. (2023, January 7). *Agoraphobia.* Mayo Clinic. Retrieved April 18, 2023, from https://www.mayoclinic.org/diseases-conditions/agoraphobia/symptoms-causes/syc-20355987

[7] Redtentwomen, B. (2018, July 03). Dear depression. Retrieved April 13, 2021, from https://redtentliving.com/2018/07/03/dear-depression/

[8] Diamond, S. A. (n.d.). *Anger disorder (Part Two): Can Bitterness become a mental disorder?* Psychology Today https://www.psychologytoday.com/us/blog/evil-deeds/200906/anger-disorder-part-two-can-bitterness-become-mental-disorder

[9] Campus Medicine. (n.d.). Clergy more likely to suffer from depression, anxiety. Duke Today. Retrieved January 3, 2022, from https://today.duke.edu/2013/08/clergydepressionnewsrelease

[10] Gesenius, W., & Tregelles, S. P. (1957). Gesenius' Hebrew and Chaldee lexicon to the Old Testament scriptures. Grand Rapids: Eerdmans.

[11] Just-world Hypothesis. The Decision Lab. (n.d.). Retrieved March 29, 2022, from https://thedecisionlab.com/biases/just-world-hypothesis

[12] Geneva College, a Christian College in Pennsylvania (PA). (2918, December 17). Geneva College Blog. The Stigma Around Mental Illness for Christians . Retrieved September 26, 2022, from https://www.geneva.edu/blog/uncategorized/stigma-mental-illness

[11] Ibid.

[14] Ibid.

[15] Ibid.

[16] Koteskey, R. L. (n.d.). Missionary care. *Depression - Missionary Care.* https://www.missionarycare.com/depression.html.

[17] Ibid.

[18]Gruver, D. (2021, February 26). *Charles Spurgeon Knew it was Possible to be Faithful and Depressed.* ChristianityToday.com. https://www.christianitytoday.com/ct/2021/february-web-only/diana-gruver-companions-darkness-spurgeon-depression.html

[19] Gruver, D. (2020). *Companions in the Darkness: Seven saints who struggled with depression and doubt* (Kindle Edition). IVP, an imprint of InterVarsity Press.

[20] Ibid.

[21] Mintle, Linda. "Can You Pray Away Mental Illness?" Can You Pray Away Mental Illness? CBN, June 7, 2017. https://www1.cbn.com/familymatters/can-you-pray-away-mental-illness

[22] Ibid.

[23] Jones, D. E., Park, J. S., Gamby, K., Bigelow, T. M., Mersha, T. B., & Folger, A. T. (2021, February 26). Mental Health Epigenetics: A Primer with implications for counselors. The Professional Counselor. Retrieved September 27, 2022, from https://tpcjournal.nbcc.org/mental-health-epigenetics-a-primer-with-implications-for-counselors/

[24] *How growing up with alcoholic parents affects children.* Addiction Center. (2023, January 9). Retrieved January 10, 2023, from https://www.addictioncenter.com/alcohol/growing-up-alcoholic-parents-affects-children/

[25] Jane Simmons. Graceworks Counseling Center of Green Acres Baptist Church. Tyler Texas.

[26] Kluger, Jeffrey. "What to Know about the CIA's Conclusion That Covid-19 Came from a Lab." Time, January 27, 2025. https://time.com/7210348/covid-19-cia-lab-leak-conclusion/.

[27] Yancey, P. (1988). What If. In Disappointment With God (pp. 49–49). essay, Walker & Company.

[28] MediLexicon International. (n.d.). *Chronic stress: Symptoms, health effects, and how to manage it.* Medical News Today https://www.addictioncenter.com/alcohol/growing-up-alcoholic-parents-affects-children/

[29] https://en.wikipedia.org/wiki/Holmes_and_Rahe_stress_scale

[30] https://www.stress.org/holmes-rahe-stress-inventory

[31] Pruett, B. and B. (2012, March 23). *Just how stressed are missionaries (and what can we do about it)?: Brian and Bailey Pruett.* Brian and Bailey Pruett | Serving in the Philippines with Aviation. Retrieved April 18, 2023, from https://blogs.ethnos360.org/brian-pruett/2012/03/23/just-how-stressed-are-missionaries-and-what-can-we-do-about-it/

[32] *Recognizing Stress.* intermountainhealthcare.org. (n.d.). https://intermountainhealthcare.org/services/wellness-preventive-medicine/live-well/feel-well/recognizing-stress/

[33] Ducharme, J. (2022, March 8). Watching war unfold on social media affects mental health. Time. Retrieved March 8, 2022, from https://time.com/6155630/ukraine-war-social-media-mental-health/

[34] Ibid.

[35] Edwards, E. (2022, October 14). Taking a break from the news can improve mental health, study finds. NBCNews.com. Retrieved October 15, 2022, from https://www.nbcnews.com/health/health-news/taking-break-news-can-improve-mental-health-study-finds-rcna51954

[36] Grammarist. (n.d.). Retrieved January 7, 2022, from https://grammarist.com/heteronyms/wound-vs-wound/

[37] Matthews, T., Danese, A., Wertz, J., Ambler, A., Kelly, M., Diver, A., Caspi, A., Moffitt, T. E., & Arseneault, L. (2015, March). Social isolation and mental health at primary and secondary school entry:

A longitudinal cohort study. Journal of the American Academy of Child and Adolescent Psychiatry.
 Retrieved March 8, 2022, from   https://www.ncbi.nlm.nih.gov/pmc/articles/PMC4733108/
[38] Wikimedia Foundation. (2022, September 28). Epigenetics. Wikipedia. Retrieved September 29, 2022,
from https://en.wikipedia.org/wiki/Epigenetics
[39] Strand, M. A., Pinkston, L. M., Chen, A. I., & Richardson, J. W. (2015). Mental health of Cross-
 Cultural HEALTHCARE MISSIONARIES. Journal of Psychology and Theology, 43(4), 283-
 293. doi:10.1177/009164711504300406
[40] I Kings 17-19
[41] Bonk, J. J., Jennings, J. N., Kim, J., & Lee, J. H. (Eds.). (2019). Missionaries, Mental Health, &
 Accountability Support Systems in Churches and Agencies. Littleton, CO: William Carey
 Publisher.
[42] Ibid.
[43] Ibid.
[44] Felman, T. (n.d.). An Unexpected Leader: A Psychiatric Analysis of King Saul [Scholarly project].
[45] Gruver, Diana. Companions in the Darkness. InterVarsity Press. Kindle Edition.
[46] Ibid.
[47] Ibid
[48] Ibid.
[49] Luther to Philip Melanchthon, October 27, 1527, in Smith and Jacobs, Luther's Correspondence, 2:419. As found in
Gruver, Diana. Companions in the Darkness . InterVarsity Press. Kindle Edition.
[50] Ibid. Gruver, Diana. Companions in the Darkness . InterVarsity Press. Kindle Edition.
[51] Luther to Jerome Weller, July 1530, in Letters of Spiritual Counsel, 85-87. Gruver, Diana.
Companions in the Darkness . InterVarsity Press. Kindle Edition.
[52] Luther, Letters of Spiritual Counsel, 95. Gruver, Diana. Companions in the Darkness . InterVarsity
Press. Kindle Edition.
[53] Charles Haddon Spurgeon, "The Exaltation of Christ," preached on November 2, 1856, New Park
Street Pulpit Vol.,
 https://www.spurgeon.org/resource-library/sermons/the-exaltation-of-christ/
[54] Carr , S. (n.d.). Charles Haddon Spurgeon and his struggle with depression. Place For Truth. Retrieved
November 3, 2021, from   https://www.placefortruth.org/blog/charles-haddon-spurgeon-and-his-
struggle-with-depression
[55] "A New Leaf for the New Year," preached on December 27, 1864, Metropolitan Tabernacle Pulpit
Vol. 42.
[56] Gruver, Diana. Companions in the Darkness . InterVarsity Press. Kindle Edition.
[57] Spurgeon, C. H. (1885, April 16). The cause and cure of a wounded spirit. The Spurgeon Center.
Retrieved November 3, 2021, from   https://www.spurgeon.org/resource-library/sermons/the-cause-
and-cure-of-a-wounded-spirit/#flipbook/.
[58] Platt, D. (2018, July 23). Lottie Moon: The long shadow of a tiny missionary giant. IMB. Retrieved
April 4, 2022, from https://www.imb.org/2018/07/23/lottie-moon-story/
[59] Ruth A. Tucker, From Jerusalem to Irian Jaya: A Biographical History of Christian Missions (Grand
Rapids, MI: Zondervan, 1983), p. 235.
[60] Gruver, Diana. Companions in the Darkness.
[61] Mother Teresa, Come Be My Light, 186-87. This is part of a prayer enclosed with   a letter to Father
Picachy dated July 3, 1959. She felt God wanted her to reveal everything to him about her interior state.
As quoted in Gruver, Diana. Companions in the Darkness. InterVarsity Press. Kindle Edition.
[62] Anne Windermere, A. (2012, February 20). 7 presidents who battled depression - symptoms -
 depression - healthcentral. 7 Presidents Who Battled Depression. Retrieved January 6, 2023,
 from https://www.healthcentral.com/article/7-presidents-who-battled-depression

[63] Strand, M. A., Pinkston, L. M., Chen, A. I., & Richardson, J. W. (2015). Mental health of Cross-Cultural HEALTHCARE MISSIONARIES. *Journal of Psychology and Theology, 43*(4), 283-293. doi:10.1177/009164711504300406
Respondents reported an average of 11 years of field experience, with 41.2% reporting that they intended to serve in cross-cultural healthcare missions until retirement. Of those who responded, 67.7% were physicians, 17% were nurses, and 15.3% served in other health-related areas. Mean age of respondents was 48 years (range: 24–85); 49.9% of respondents were male and 50.1% were female. All the participants in this study were career missionaries employed by organizations whose primary purpose was selecting and training personnel for long term cross-cultural service.

[64] Duke University. (2013, August 27). Clergy more likely to suffer from depression, anxiety. Duke Today. Retrieved April 4, 2022, from https://today.duke.edu/2013/08/clergydepressionnewsrelease#

[65] Megan Briggs, M. B. (2020, August 29). Why are pastors depressed? A look at the research. ChurchLeaders. Retrieved April 4, 2022, from https://churchleaders.com/news/359562-why-are-pastors-depressed-a-look-at-the-research.html

[66] Lovett, I. (2020, January 20). It's like I got kicked out of my family.' churches struggle with mental health in the ranks. The Wall Street Journal. Retrieved April 4, 2022, from https://www.wsj.com/articles/its-like-i-got-kicked-out-of-my-family-churches-struggle-with-mental-health-in-the-ranks-11579547221

[67] Brennan, D. Medical Reviewer (2021, October 1). What are the 4 major causes of depression? MedicineNet. Retrieved April 4, 2022, from https://www.medicinenet.com/what_are_4_major_causes_of_depression/article.htm

[68] Depression (major depressive disorder). (2018, February 03). Retrieved April 22, 2021, from https://www.mayoclinic.org/diseases-conditions/depression/symptoms-causes/syc-20356007

[69] Ingram, C., & Johnson, B. C. (2010). *Overcoming emotions that destroy: practical help for those angry feelings that ruin relationships.* Baker Books.

[70] Ibid, 29.

[71] SoP. (2021, April 4). *Prefrontal cortex.* The Science of Psychotherapy. Retrieved April 10, 2023, from https://www.thescienceofpsychotherapy.com/prefrontal-cortex/

[72] Hathaway, W. R., & Newton, B. W. (2022, June 5). *Neuroanatomy, Prefrontal Cortex - Statpearls - NCBI bookshelf.* Neuroanatomy, Prefrontal Cortex. Retrieved April 4, 2023, from https://www.ncbi.nlm.nih.gov/books/NBK499919/

[73] GoodTherapy. (n.d.). Prefrontal Cortex. GoodTherapy.org Therapy Blog. Retrieved May 28, 2022, from https://www.goodtherapy.org/blog/psychpedia/prefrontal-cortex

[74] John Hopkins Medicine. (2021, July 14). Brain Anatomy and How the Brain Works. Johns Hopkins Medicine. Retrieved May 28, 2022, from https://www.hopkinsmedicine.org/health/conditions-and-diseases/anatomy-of-the-brain

[75] Sukel, K. (2019, July 28). *Beyond Emotion: Understanding the Amygdala's Role in Memory.* Dana Foundation. https://dana.org/article/beyond-emotion-understanding-the-amygdalas-role-in-memory/.

[76] Young, A. (2020, May 8). *The upstairs and downstairs of The brain: Part one.* Kids That Go. Retrieved April 10, 2023, from https://kidsthatgo.com/upstairs-and-downstairs-brain-part-one/

[77] Ingram, C., & Johnson, B. C. (2010). *Overcoming emotions that destroy: practical help for those angry feelings that ruin relationships.* Baker Books.

[78] Young, A. (2020, May 8). *The upstairs and downstairs of The brain: Part one*. Kids That Go. Retrieved April 10, 2023, from https://kidsthatgo.com/upstairs-and-downstairs-brain-part-one/

[79] Karmin, A. (2017). The Physiology of Anger. In *Anger management workbook for men: take control of your anger and master your emotions* (pp. 45–60). essay, Althea Press, 4-47.

[80] Sahu, A., Gupta, P., & Chatterjee, B. (2014, January). *Depression is More Than Just Sadness: A Case of Excessive Anger and Its Management in Depression*. Indian journal of psychological medicine. https://www.ncbi.nlm.nih.gov/pmc/articles/PMC3959025/.

[81] Lewis L. Judd, M. D. (2013, November 1). *Overt Irritability/Anger in Unipolar MDEs*. JAMA Psychiatry. https://jamanetwork.com/journals/jamapsychiatry/fullarticle/1737169.

[82] Ingram, C., & Johnson, 15.

[83] *Health Costs Of Anger*. Mental Help Health Costs Of Anger Comments. (n.d.). https://www.mentalhelp.net/anger/health-costs/.

[84] Ingram, C., & Johnson.

[85] Thomson Reuters. (n.d.). How to avoid missed expectations. How to avoid missed expectations | Thomson Reuters. Retrieved April 5, 2022, from
https://legal.thomsonreuters.com/en/insights/articles/avoiding-missed-expectations

[86] Ibid, 89.

[87] Ingram , C. (2019). *Rage: Understanding the Monster Within (Part 1) James 1:19-20*. Over Coming Emotions that Destroy. Retrieved September 9, 2021, from
https://messagenotes.livingontheedge.org/Overcoming-Emotions-That-Destroy.pdf.

[88] *G4088 - Pikria - Strong's Greek lexicon (KJV)*. Blue Letter Bible. (n.d.). Retrieved September 16, 2021, from https://www.blueletterbible.org/lexicon/g4088/kjv/tr/0-1/.

[89] *Wrath - vine's expository dictionary of NT words -*. StudyLight.org. (n.d.). Retrieved September 16, 2021, from https://www.studylight.org/dictionaries/eng/ved/w/wrath.html.

[90] *G3709 - orgē - strong's Greek lexicon (KJV)*. Blue Letter Bible. (n.d.). Retrieved September 16, 2021, from https://www.blueletterbible.org/lexicon/g3709/kjv/tr/0-1/.

[91] *G988 - blasphēmia - Strong's Greek lexicon (KJV)*. Blue Letter Bible. (n.d.). Retrieved September 16, 2021, from https://www.blueletterbible.org/lexicon/g988/kjv/tr/0-1/.

[92] https://www.blueletterbible.org/lexicon/g5543/nlt/mgnt/0-1/

[93] Ibid.

[94] Ingram , C. (2019). *Rage: Understanding the Monster Within (Part 1) James 1:19-20*.

[95] Diamond, S. A. (n.d.). *Anger disorder (Part Two): Can Bitterness become a mental disorder?* Psychology Today. https://www.psychologytoday.com/us/blog/evil-deeds/200906/anger-disorder-part-two-can-bitterness-become-mental-disorder.

[96] Ibid.

[97] Kittel, G., & Bromiley, G. (1967). μιαίνω. In THEOLOGICAL dictionary of the New Testament: VOL. 4. edited by G. Kittel ; edited and translated by G.W. BROMILEY (Vol. 4, Ser. Reprinted September 1978, pp. 644–647). essay, WM B. Eerdmans Publishing Co.

[98] *G3392 - miainō - strong's greek lexicon (kjv)*. Blue Letter Bible. (n.d.). https://www.blueletterbible.org/lexicon/g3392/kjv/tr/0-1/.

[99] Kittel, G., & Bromiley, G. (1967). μιαίνω, 646.

[100] Ibid.

[101] Fuller, J. R. (2014, October 5). *Bitterness Is It Blocked Anger or A Real Mental Disorder?* CBT Therapist NYC | NYC Psychologist | Dr. J. Ryan Fuller. https://jryanfuller.com/treatment/anger-treatment/bitterness-is-it-blocked-anger-or-a-real-mental-disorder/.

[102] Hostetler, B., Hamlin, R., & Ciancanelli, S. (2022, June 28). *7 Prayers of Release*. Guideposts. Retrieved February 22, 2023, from https://guideposts.org/prayer/inspirational-prayers/7-prayers-of-release/

[103] McLean Hospital. (2021, February 10). The social Dilemma: Social media and your mental health. Retrieved April 14, 2021, from https://www.mcleanhospital.org/essential/it-or-not-social-medias-affecting-your-mental-health

[104] Mir, E., Novas, C., & Meg, M. (2021, March 17). Social media and ADOLESCENTS' and young Adults' mental health. Retrieved April 14, 2021, from https://www.center4research.org/social-media-affects-mental-health/

[105] AnnaVannuccia, Kaitlin M. Flannery, Christine McCauley Ohannessianac. "Social Media Use and Anxiety in Emerging Adults." Journal of Affective Disorders. Elsevier, October 3, 2016. https://www.sciencedirect.com/science/article/abs/pii/S0165032716309442.

[106] "Social Media and Mental Health." HelpGuide.org. HelpGuide. Accessed December 22, 2022. https://www.helpguide.org/articles/mental-health/social-media-and-mental-health.htm.

[107] The state of mental health in America. (2021). Retrieved April 14, 2021, from https://www.mhanational.org/issues/state-mental-health-america/

[108] *Philippians 4 : English Standard Version (ESV)*. Blue Letter Bible. (n.d.). Retrieved February 24, 2023, from https://www.blueletterbible.org/esv/phl/4/8/t_conc_1107008

[109] Ibid.

[110] Ibid.

[111] Ibid.

[112] Ibid.

[113] Ibid.

[114] Ibid.

[115] Ibid.

[116] "Social Media and Mental Health." HelpGuide.org

[117] Mayo Foundation for Medical Education and Research. (2020, September 15). *Can mindfulness exercises help me?* Mayo Clinic. https://www.mayoclinic.org/healthy-lifestyle/consumer-health/in-depth/mindfulness-exercises/art-20046356.

[118] *Christian Virtue & Mindfulness*. THE MINDFUL CHRISTIAN. (n.d.). Retrieved April 5, 2023, from https://www.themindfulchristian.com/christian_virtue.html

[119] Focus on the Family. (2023, February 8). *Mindfulness: A Christian Approach*. MINDFULNESS: A CHRISTIAN APPROACH. Retrieved April 11, 2023, from https://www.focusonthefamily.com/family-qa/mindfulness-a-christian-approach/

[120] Christian Virtue & Mindfulness. THE MINDFUL CHRISTIAN. (n.d.). Retrieved March 9, 2022, from https://www.themindfulchristian.com/christian_virtue.html

[121] Mayo Foundation for Medical Education and Research. (2021, July 29). Stress relief from laughter? it's no joke. Mayo Clinic. Retrieved December 10, 2021, from https://www.mayoclinic.org/healthy-lifestyle/stress-management/in-depth/stress-relief/art-20044456.

[122] Ibid.

[123] Ibid.

[124] Starr, M. (2022, March 22). It's official: NASA confirms we've found 5,000   worlds outside the solar system. ScienceAlert. Retrieved March 24, 2022, from https://www.sciencealert.com/it-s-official-we-have-now-confirmed-over-5-000-worlds-outside-the-solar-system

[125] G5479 - chara - strong's Greek lexicon (KJV). Blue Letter Bible. (n.d.). Retrieved December 10, 2021, from   https://www.blueletterbible.org/lexicon/g5479/kjv/tr/0-1/.

[126] *Forgiveness: Your health depends on it*. Forgiveness: Your Health Depends on It | Johns Hopkins Medicine. (2021, November 1). Retrieved January 14, 2023, from https://www.hopkinsmedicine.org/health/wellness-and-prevention/forgiveness-your-health-depends-on-it

[127] McNeill, B. (2017, April 24). After four decades, Everett Worthington, leading expert on forgiveness, set to retire from VCU's Department of Psychology. VCU News. Retrieved June 6, 2022, from https://news.vcu.edu/article/After_four_decades_Everett_Worthington_leading_expert_on_forgiveness

[128] Ibid.

[129] Weir, K. (2017, January). Forgiveness can improve mental and physical health - Vol 48, No. 1. Monitor on Psychology. Retrieved February 8, 2022, from https://www.apa.org/monitor/2017/01/ce-corner

[130] Ibid.

[131] Mayo Clinic Staff. (2020, November 13). Why is it so easy to hold a grudge? Mayo Clinic. Retrieved February 8, 2022, from https://www.mayoclinic.org/healthy-lifestyle/adult-health/in-depth/forgiveness/art-20047692

[132] Weir, K. (2017, January).

[133] *Forgiveness. Ephesians 4:32 | Videos | YouVersion*. YouVersion Bible. Accessed December 17, 2022. https://www.bible.com/en/videos/37817?orientation=portrait&utm_content=story_clip&utm_medium=share&utm_source=yvapp.

[134] Ibid.

[135] Wikimedia Foundation. (2021, December 6). Don Quixote. Wikipedia. Retrieved December 16, 2021, from https://en.wikipedia.org/wiki/Don_Quixote

[136] Literature Network. (n.d.). About this translation. The Literature Network: Online classic literature, poems, and quotes. Essays & Summaries. Retrieved December 16, 2021, from http://www.online-literature.com/cervantes/don_quixote/12/

[137] Ma, L. (Ed.). (2016, April 16). 5 Ways to Stop Your Racing Thoughts | Psychology Today. 5 Ways to Stop Your Racing Thoughts. Retrieved February 7, 2022, from   https://www.psychologytoday.com/us/blog/women-s-mental-health-matters/201604/5-ways-stop-your-racing-thoughts

[138] Ibid.

[139] https://www.blueletterbible.org/lexicon/h5564/kjv/wlc/0-1/

[140] U.S. Department of Health and Human Services. (n.d.). Chronic illness and   mental health: Recognizing and treating depression. National Institute of Mental Health. Retrieved November 21, 2021, from   https://www.nimh.nih.gov/health/publications/chronic-illness-mental-health.

[141] Physical Health and Mental Health. Mental Health Foundation. (2021, July 20). Retrieved November 21, 2021, from https://www.mentalhealth.org.uk/a-to-z/p/physical-health-and-mental-health.

[142] Ibid.

[143] Seltzer, L. F. (2016, August 24). Self-absorption: The root of all (psychological) evil... Self-Absorption: The Root of All (Psychological) Evil? Retrieved December 23, 2021, https://www.psychologytoday.com/us/blog/evolution-the-self/201608/self-absorption-the-root-all-psychological-evil

[144] Copenhaver, M. B. (2014). Jesus is the question: The 307 questions Jesus asked   and the 3 he answered. Abingdon Press.

[145] Ibid.

[146] Jackson, Dory. "Michael J. Fox Says 'Gratitude Makes Optimism Sustainable' While Living with Parkinson's Disease." Peoplemag. PEOPLE, November 30, 2021. https://people.com/tv/michael-j-fox-gratitude-makes-optimism-sustainable-parkinsons-disease/.

[147] Kaufman, S. B. (2020, June 29). Unraveling the Mindset of Victimhood. Scientific American. Retrieved March 28, 2022, from https://www.scientificamerican.com/article/unraveling-the-mindset-of-victimhood/

[148] Ibid.

www.ingramcontent.com/pod-product-compliance
Lightning Source LLC
Chambersburg PA
CBHW071119280326
41935CB00010B/1060